BUILDING *CONFIANZA*

GLOBAL LATIN/O AMERICAS

Frederick Luis Aldama and Lourdes Torres, Series Editors

BUILDING *CONFIANZA*

EMPOWERING LATINOS/AS
THROUGH TRANSCULTURAL
HEALTH CARE COMMUNICATION

Dalia Magaña

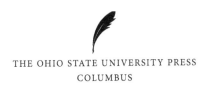

THE OHIO STATE UNIVERSITY PRESS
COLUMBUS

Library of Congress Cataloging-in-Publication Data
Names: Magaña, Dalia, author.
Title: Building confianza : empowering Latinos/as through transcultural health care communication / Dalia Magaña.
Other titles: Global Latin/o Americas.
Description: Columbus : The Ohio State University Press, [2021] | Series: Global Latin/o Americas | Includes bibliographical references and index. | Summary: "Draws on systemic functional linguistics discourse analysis to analyze how Latino/a patients narrate their experiences in psychiatric intake interviews and explores the importance of transcultural competency in health care"—Provided by publisher.
Identifiers: LCCN 2021018797 | ISBN 9780814214817 (cloth) | ISBN 0814214819 (cloth) | ISBN 9780814281635 (ebook) | ISBN 081428163X (ebook)
Subjects: LCSH: Communication in medicine. | Language and medicine. | Transcultural medical care. | Hispanic Americans—Medical care. | Spanish language—Discourse analysis. | Medical care—Cross-cultural studies. | Discourse analysis, Narrative. | Linguistic analysis (Linguistics)
Classification: LCC P302.7 .M34 2021 | DDC 610.1/4—dc23
LC record available at https://lccn.loc.gov/2021018797

Cover design by Larry Nozik
Text design by Stuart Rodriguez
Type set in Minion Pro

C O N T E N T S

List of Illustrations   vii

Acknowledgments   ix

Prologue   xi

CHAPTER 1   Communicating with Latino/as in Health Care: Language
              Barriers and Transcultural Competence   1

CHAPTER 2   Psychiatric Interviews as a Genre and Patients' Narratives   23

CHAPTER 3   *Hacer Plática*: Small Talk Subgenres   49

CHAPTER 4   Register of the Psychiatric Interview: Interlocutors,
              Power, and Solidarity   67

CHAPTER 5   Translanguaging in Health Care Interactions   89

CHAPTER 6   Expressing Verbal Modality and Other Politeness
              Strategies in Psychiatric Interviews   107

CHAPTER 7   Conclusions: Spanish and Transcultural Discourse in
              Health, Teaching, and Research   125

Appendix I   *Summary of Patients' Backgrounds*   139

Appendix II   *Sample of a Complete Interview*   143

References   157

Index   169

ILLUSTRATIONS

FIGURES

FIGURE 1	Language, genre, register, and cultural constructs	14
FIGURE 2	Deviations from short responses	44
FIGURE 3	Formality language levels of affect, frequency of contact, and power	76

TABLES

TABLE 1	Register variable and language metafunctions	13
TABLE 2	Summary of generic components of psychiatric interviews, subgenres, and function	27
TABLE 3	Colloquialisms and standard synonyms	72
TABLE 4	Patients' descriptions of depression and anxiety symptoms	74
TABLE 5	Patient questions in studies on medical consultations and sample size	83
TABLE 6	Words spoken by doctor and patients	84
TABLE 7	Interruptions by doctor and patients	85
TABLE 8	Total code-switches by doctor and patients	94
TABLE 9	Code-switching categories used by doctor and patients	94

ACKNOWLEDGMENTS

I owe gratitude to many people for making this book possible.

First, I am grateful to the patients who gave consent for this study and the researchers who were a part of the original study. The health stories of patients have offered me light through their admirable resilience.

Along the book's journey, I have counted on the generous support of many brilliant scholars.

I am indebted to Glenn Martínez for paving the way in the field of medical Spanish and Latinx health discourse, which has opened opportunities to many linguists and the communities they serve. Cecilia Colombi, one of my earliest mentors, has also created intellectual spaces for linguistic theory that connects to local bilinguals in meaningful ways. Both have been strong advocates of my work and have had a profound influence on my thinking. I am sincerely thankful to Glenn, Cecilia, and Alberto Odor for generously offering their advice during initial planning and for connecting me to the people and resources that helped bring this book to light. I also thank them, along with Julia Menard Warwick, for carefully commenting on the entire manuscript and offering robust feedback, which improved the book's argument. They all encouraged me with their belief in the project's value.

Adam Schwartz, Roberto Heredia, and Robert Train have also supported my work and offered me guidance when I have presented parts of this book. The *International Journal of the Linguistic Association of the Southwest* published an early version of chapter 3 on small talk. I also published sections of chapter 6 in *Communication & Medicine*. I am grateful to the journals' editors and anonymous reviewers for their helpful feedback.

I owe a sincere thanks to many of my UC Merced colleagues. My department and humanities colleagues have offered me immense support (Arturo Arias, Cristián Ricci, Ignacio López-Calvo, Katie Brokaw, Kit Meyers, Manuel Martín-Rodríguez, Mario Sifuentez, Virginia Adán-Lifante, to name a few). I am also grateful to Teenie Matlock and Tanya Golash Boza for their generous mentorship and advocacy. Numerous exchanges with Whitney Pirtle and Ma Vang have helped shape my thinking. They have offered me intellectual, emotional, and writing support. I thank them for their constructive feedback on the book's opening. I also thank them, as well as Christina Lux, Denise Payan, and Lorena Alvarado, for our writing groups. Mauricio Martinez and Lorraine Ramos offered excellent research assistance, for which I am genuinely grateful.

I thank the UC Merced Center for Humanities for their generous funding to support this book.

This book benefited from several careful reviews by Kate Epstein, a gifted editor, who offered substantive editing. I owe gratitude to her for her thorough technical and stylistic comments, which helped improve the language and argument's clarity.

At The Ohio State University Press, Kristen A. Elias Rowley has been a remarkable editor-in-chief, guiding me through the publication process and offering me timely support. I am fortunate to work with such a talented editor-in-chief and team. I also thank Frederick Luis Aldama and Lourdes Torres, editors of the Global Latin/o Americas book series, for believing in this project and for their guidance. I sincerely appreciate the anonymous reviewers' effort and generosity with their time in carefully reviewing my manuscript. Their constructive comments helped enhance the quality of this manuscript and its argument.

My heartfelt thanks go to my husband, Cesar Casillas, and my children, Celeste, Damian, and Ciara, for their love, patience, and encouragement every step of the way.

I am also grateful to my mother, whose language and cultural struggles in health care inspired this book.

PROLOGUE

I began interpreting for my mother at age six. My awareness of how language and cultural differences disadvantage immigrants in the US grew naturally from interpreting for her. My mother came to San Jose, California, from a rural town in Mexico, two years before I was born, in order to financially help her mother and siblings in Mexico, and to provide basic opportunities for herself and her future children: my two younger brothers and me. A single mom, she supported us by working night shifts as a janitor, where she spoke Spanish with her boss and co-workers. Although she enrolled in adult English classes, her comprehension remained minimal. One of the reasons for her limited English comprehension is that her literacy skills in Spanish were not strong—she had to leave school at a young age and begin working. Thus, learning English based on tasks involving reading was very challenging. Her limited English has created many cultural and communication barriers in all institutional sectors, including health care. Among the most dangerous arose after a breast cancer diagnosis.

In May 2011 my mother told me that she had had a mammogram, but that she didn't have cancer. She said there was a possibility that in the future she might develop it, but that she was not worried. She mentioned that she has no family history of breast cancer. I knew that the nurse at the community clinic was bilingual, but I was still nervous. My mother mistrusts doctors and does not get regular mammograms; the test had been prompted by the nurse finding a lump during an exam. I had often seen miscommunication between her and health care providers in the years when I regularly interpreted for her, and I had seen interpreters mistreat her. She also has trouble speaking up even in Spanish, in part because of her upbringing. Her strict father taught her to defer to authority figures, and she has continued the practice. I think she is also self-conscious because she speaks a register associated with the working class. At times she has trouble understanding words associated with middle-class Spanish, including Spanish spoken in medical contexts. To me it seemed quite likely that she had cancer and that if left untreated, it would soon take her life.

I was close to taking my PhD qualifying exams and taking care of my new baby, her second grandchild, at the time, but I drove two hours to be with her at her next appointment. As it began, I could see that the doctor was visibly upset. She told me that my mother was being noncompliant, that she was not answering calls and was missing appointments. I was shocked. As I interpreted for her, the doctor explained to us that my mom did have early-stage breast cancer and recommended a lumpectomy followed by radiation.

It took a few weeks for my mother to accept her diagnosis. She told me that the word *cancer* frightened her. To her it meant being closer to death. She was also worried about having surgery because she believed that if she did have cancer, the cancer would spread throughout her body during the procedure. In general she is suspicious of doctors. She heard that there were cases where doctors performed unnecessary procedures and used people to experiment with their bodies. Maybe the doctors were making up the diagnosis.

When she finally came to terms with it, she said that God wanted her to have cancer and that she should not seek treatment. Knowing of her deep faith, I reminded her of the saying that God helps those who help themselves (*Ayúdate y Dios te ayudará*). She finally agreed to have the surgery and undergo radiation.

On the scheduled day of her surgery, a nurse attached the word *noncompliant* to my mother again. She had not had the EKG, pregnancy test, and blood test required before the surgery. I had not been at the appointment where these tests were ordered, but it was apparent to me that my mother had not fully understood the preoperative instructions. The operation had to be rescheduled for two weeks later, at which time it went ahead. Radiation therapy followed with minimal difficulty.

Months later the doctor diagnosed a recurrence and urged my mother to undergo a mastectomy. She refused at first. When I begged her to listen to her doctor, she would say that she didn't feel a lump or cancer inside her, that she didn't trust doctors. She used a simile: what would I do if a doctor wanted to amputate one of my fingers even though it looked and felt healthy? She felt her breast was healthy and that the procedure would leave her unnecessarily disfigured. It took me weeks to convince her to follow her provider's recommendation of undergoing a mastectomy, but she eventually did. While she has been in remission for years now, I am well aware of how close I came to losing her.

When I served as an instructor for basic-level Spanish during my graduate training in Hispanic linguistics at UC Davis, I gained a new perspective on why medical practitioners and interpreters had so often failed my mother. California has many Spanish-speaking communities, including my family's, yet the assigned textbook did not teach my students how to speak to any of them. The vocabulary I was teaching would have been mostly unfamiliar to my mother. It was supposed to be teaching generic, hyperstandard world Spanish, but it privileged the language of middle-class speakers, sometimes focused on Peninsular Spanish phrases and terms. Everyday vocabulary lessons included topics such as skiing, getting service at restaurants, and traveling. It clearly reflected language ideologies of how middle-class speakers use Spanish. Varieties of working-class people, those in need of language services in our immediate communities, were not included. Our students might be prepared to travel to Spain or Argentina, but they would not be able to converse with the Mexican immigrants who predominate in California.

It was explained to me that I was supposed to be preparing students for interactions across numerous Spanish speakers, that we should not limit our teaching to one variety, because Spanish is spoken across numerous countries. Indeed, Spanish in the US varies widely—Puerto Rican Spanish is most common in parts of the Midwest and the East Coast and is different from Cuban Spanish in Florida, Central American Spanish in California and the East Coast, and Mexican Spanish in the Southwest and Midwest. Yet, preparing students for study abroad in Spain or Argentina and only for speaking to middle-class people did not seem neutral, and many of my students hoped to be able to use their Spanish locally. Thus, I began to supplement course materials with colloquial Mexican Spanish and emphasized the value of local knowledge. I wanted to help prepare students for local interactions even if it contradicted some of the language ideologies of the textbook in terms of what was proper Spanish. If any of my students entered health care practice in California, they would need these lessons.

More classrooms need to teach working-class Spanish to address health care disparities that affect Latino/as across the US. But as this book describes, teaching varieties that are disregarded in language textbooks or frankly called wrong in Spanish-language classrooms is the tip of the iceberg. This book reflects on authentic interactions in health care discourse, assessing the many tools that a Mexican immigrant doctor uses to reach patients similar linguistically and culturally to my mother. In so doing, it uses linguistics as a tool to center voices of working-class Spanish speakers as recipients of health care. This book brings to light explicit awareness of what cultural and linguistic competence means during interactions between Mexican patients and a Mexican doctor across numerous real-world examples. I hope to raise awareness about how to train providers and interpreters to connect to local communities of Spanish speakers when they seek health care, a highly vulnerable and critical moment. In doing so, I hope to contribute to a more inclusive society by promoting the language and culture of Mexican-origin people in critical contexts, to ensure that immigrants like my mother receive the high-quality care and respect they deserve.

CHAPTER 1

Communicating with Latino/as in Health Care

Language Barriers and Transcultural Competence

Fue entrando el doctor con los papeles con los resultados del análisis y me dice, "No tienes cancer." "Ay," dije. "¿Perdón?" le dije, "ése [análisis] era para ver si tenía cáncer y ¿por qué no me dijeron?" ¿Qué es una biopsia? No, no me dijeron. Es necesario decirme. Soy yo y es mi cuerpo.

The doctor entered with the paperwork with the results of the analysis and says to me, "You don't have cancer." "Wow" I said. "Excuse me?" I told him, "that [analysis] was to see if I had cancer and why didn't they tell me?" What is a biopsy? They didn't tell me. It's necessary to tell me. This is about me and it is my body. (Milagros, a Mexican woman in her fifties living in California's Central Valley)

—Magaña 2020

MILAGROS SHARED WITH ME a clear case of miscommunication in health care. She said that she had felt worse than disempowered when she received a biopsy without any culturally appropriate explanation of biopsies; she was shocked and frustrated when her doctor gave her the good news that she didn't have cancer. She said, rightly, that she has a right to understand procedures involving her own body (Magaña 2020). Miscommunication in health care is a frequent occurrence that jeopardizes the health of Spanish-speaking Latino/as.[1] The problem is not necessarily a lack of interpreters. President Bill Clinton's Executive Order 13166, "Improving Access to Services for Persons with Limited English Proficiency," had required large health care organization in regions with significant proportions of limited English proficient persons to provide interpreter services for non-English-speaking patients since 2000 (Martínez 2008). For Californians, SB 853, the Health Care Language Assis-

---

1. In this book I use *Latino/a* as an inclusive term to refer to people with heritage in Latin America. When used as an adjective, as in Latino health, it is meant to be gender neutral. I recognize the progressive use of Latinx but do not use it here because it is not a term that patients in this study use to identify themselves.

tance Act, has required health insurance plans to provide interpreters and translated materials since 2009. However, interpreter-mediated interactions have significant limitations (Davidson 2001). Because of these limitations, interventions from bicultural and bilingual family members, health promoters, or medical personnel whom patients trust have been shown to improve outcomes.

Providers who speak the same language as patients are far superior to interpreters (Ngo-Metzger et al. 2007). Yet, linguistic competency alone does not suffice for optimal care; transcultural competence, meaning knowledge of the symbolic value of language and the ability to translate information culturally, is just as critical (Kramsch 2010). This transcultural knowledge may entail awareness of patients' sociopolitical situations in the US. For instance, it is crucial for providers to be aware of the context of Latino/a patients in relation to immigration history, structural inequalities, and racist attitudes and policies that affect many of these groups today, as all of these factors contribute to health disparities (Y. Flores 2013). Latino/as in the US face higher rates of cervical cancer and HIV and AIDS, musculoskeletal diseases, and pesticide poisoning, and a higher risk of dying of diabetes than their non-Hispanic white counterparts (De la Torre and Estrada 2015).

Beyond language competency and cultural competency, doctors need to know how to answer the following questions across numerous interaction types: How do providers and patients build trust and solidarity with each other? How do doctors use their cultural and sociopolitical knowledge to get patients to tell their health stories? How do patients discuss and understand their illness? How do they talk about their health situations? These questions have been long neglected. This book uses a linguistic lens to examine authentic medical interactions to address these questions.

In so doing, this study builds on linguistics studies considering the intersection between medicine and language that have significantly advanced our knowledge regarding medical discourse and have influenced more patient-centered care. However, most research has focused on English-language interactions. Studies on Spanish-language interactions generally were undertaken in contexts where Spanish is the majority language (Cordella 2004; Delbene 2004). The US health care system is primarily geared toward serving English-speakers (Timmins 2002).

Drawing on systemic functional linguistics (SFL)—a discourse analysis theory founded by M. A. K. Halliday (1978)—and sociolinguistics perspectives, this book provides linguistic insights into how rural Mexican patients narrate their experiences during an intake psychiatric interview and how they negotiate aspects of the roles related to social expectations and power dynamics. Use of SFL allows multiple levels of discourse analysis to illustrate the genre (i.e., cultural context), register (i.e., situational factors influencing communication, including the relationship between interlocutors), and interpersonal language (with an emphasis on verbal modality and politeness) in psychiatric interviews.

This book examines how one doctor, whom I call Dr. Ortiz, and twenty-three patients negotiate language and cultural knowledge. It looks, for example, at the case of a patient in his mid-forties who tells Dr. Ortiz that he is not taking his medication because he read the word *drug* on the label and understood the term to mean *illegal drug*. Spanish-language skills do not guarantee that a doctor will know that in the patient's rural Spanish variety, *drogas* typically means *illegal drugs*.

Beyond sociolinguistic awareness, I find that doctors must create interpersonal relationships that will help generate trust and empower patients. Small talk, humor, self-disclosure, and informal language (e.g., code-switching and colloquialisms) are key tools for creating such relationships. Here again, language skills are important: being sociolinguistically informed and having advanced language skills permits providers to move from medical registers to informal ones to make interpersonal connections with patients and, as a result, gain their trust and communicate more clearly about their health issues.

This study offers interventions for improving health care communication using data from authentic doctor–patient interviews with a doctor who is both sociolinguistically informed and a native speaker of Spanish. Few studies have addressed Spanish-language interactions between Latino/as and their doctors, despite the growth of the US Latino/a population; thus, this study addresses a significant gap in the literature. Same-language and same-culture models of doctor and patient interactions are crucial for training doctors and improving the quality of health care for language-minority patients in the US. I propose that practitioners can communicate acceptance and respect for the patient's language by having sociolinguistic awareness and demonstrating transcultural knowledge of the patient's culture, all of which is revealed by the language choices made during medical interactions.

Transcultural Competence

This project builds on the concept of transcultural competence. Transcultural communication in the medical context I study entails knowledge of the language, socialization, cultural values, sociopolitical history, and practices of patients (Kramsch 2010). The exchanges analyzed are not merely between cultures, as the term *intercultural* may suggest, but instead across cultures in a society where the Spanish language plays a complex role because of its social and political history. Further, transcultural communication requires familiarity with patients' socialization practices, meaning knowledge of their social, linguistic, and cultural systems and the issues that minority groups in the US face concerning language, power, and society (Martínez 2011; Martínez and Schwartz 2012). Therefore, transcultural competency presupposes sociolinguistic awareness and advanced proficiency in Spanish that enables practitioners to connect to patients in local communities (Colombi and Magaña 2013).

Equally as important as formal and technical registers of Spanish, informal and colloquial registers aid practitioners in their communication with local communities. One problem is that patients' varieties are often stigmatized and silenced in educational materials (Martínez and Schwartz 2012). This compounds the vulnerability of patients already disadvantaged in health care because of their literacy limitations, socioeconomic status, cultural and language barriers, and education levels.

This book responds to the urgent need for research on doctor–patient interactions that provide a specific description of transcultural communication, delineating it in explicit terms in a specific health context. The data for this study consist of intake psychiatric interviews conducted in Spanish in rural California. The stigmatization of psychiatric disorders and of seeking mental health care makes psychiatric interviews a high-stakes context for discourse analysis. The psychiatric interviews analyzed share similarities with medical interviews in other health settings. However, they differ from a routine consultation, for example, given the in-depth answers patients may offer about their clinical and sociodevelopmental history, making this context particularly rich for analyzing health care interactions, as discussed in chapter 2. This interdisciplinary work speaks to scholars in linguistics and health communication. The study thus opens a window into how doctors and patients who share the same language and ethnicity negotiate traditionally taboo topics.

In sum, this book has two primary aims. First, it describes the language of Spanish psychiatric interviews in the US with a focus on medical narratives and interpersonal language. Second, it reveals transcultural strategies that Dr. Ortiz uses to adapt the interview to the needs of his patients. This book explores the culturally embedded language choices that one doctor makes and the strategies he uses to obtain health information from patients in culturally and linguistically sensitive ways.

Latino/as, Language, and Health in the US

Latino/as[2] are the largest minority group in the US, accounting for 17 percent of the population (US Census Bureau 2016). Of all Latino groups, people of Mexican descent are the majority (64 percent), and most are concentrated in California and Texas. California has 15.5 million Hispanic residents, the largest Latino population of any state in the country (US Census Bureau 2018). The state is also unique in having a minority-majority population: Hispanics or Latino/as are 39.1 percent of the state's population and growing (US Census Bureau 2018). The Spanish language plays an essential role in communication among Latino families: 73 percent of Latino/as over the age of five speak Spanish at home (US Census Bureau 2015). Almost a third of this group is not fluent in English (US Census Bureau 2016).

Language barriers have a direct impact on health care and the health outcomes and disparities that Latino/as face. Research shows that discordant communication between doctors and patients who speak different languages leads to lengthier hospital stays and a higher incidence of medical errors and risks to patients, and to patients receiving less health education, having lower medical instruction comprehension, and experiencing greater dissatisfaction with the quality of interpersonal care (Elderkin-Thompson et al. 2001; G. Flores 2006; Hernández et al. 2011; Lee et al. 2002; Ngo-Metzger et al. 2007; Perez-Stable et al. 1997). Patients with limited command of English are less likely to use primary and preventive care and public health services and are more likely to use emergency departments, where they receive fewer services than their English-dominant counterparts (Youdelman 2008).

The mental health picture reveals numerous disparities. Research has found that structural inequalities contribute to depression among Mexicans (Y. Flores 2013; Lackey 2008). One study found that Mexicans attribute depression to issues of migration, separation from loved ones due to immigration, racial and socioeconomic discrimination and harassment, inequalities in pay, and language barriers in the US (Lackey 2008). Latino/as have a prevalence of depression similar to non-Latino whites but are less likely to receive diagnosis and treatment than non-Latino whites or to return for a second appointment after an initial visit to a psychologist (Alegría et al. 2008; Dingfelder 2005; Wassertheil-Smoller et al. 2014). Colon et al. (2013) attribute the underdiag-

---

2. Latino/as living in the US include groups diverse in ethnicity (e.g., Cuban, Salvadoran, Puerto Rican, Mexican), race, socioeconomic status, and language levels in Spanish, English, or an indigenous language. This book examines medical interviews with people of Mexican origin living in rural California, and I do not suggest that all Latino/as are similar to this group.

nosis of Latino/as in part to the lack of culturally adapted and effective assessment tools. Immigration and acculturation and low socioeconomic status and education levels predict depression, and these factors disproportionately affect Latino/as (López and Carrillo 2001).

Latino/as also face disparities in treating mental health. A study of 16,000 participants across Latino groups found depressive symptoms in 27 percent of respondents. But only 5 percent were taking antidepressants (Wassertheil-Smoller et al. 2014), which contrasts with 13.6 percent of non-Hispanic whites with similar symptoms (Pratt et al. 2011). Similarly, Spanish-dominant Latino/as are less likely to obtain and engage in mental health care (Bauer et al. 2010). Although a study of Latino participants reports that antidepressants alleviate symptoms (Cabassa et al. 2008), research suggests that Latino/as underuse medication because of fear of addiction and other harmful side effects as well as a stigmatized view of mental health issues (Interian et al. 2011). Stigmatization of depression among Latino/as creates concerns about judgment from friends and family and pressure to manage the disease without help (Uebelacker et al. 2012). One study on women, including Latinas, found that participants with depression had even higher levels of stigmatized views of depression than those without (Nadeem et al. 2007). Another study identifies *vergüenza*—embarrassment/shame—as a particular risk among Latino/as who experience depression (Marquez and Ramírez García 2013).

For Spanish-dominant Latino/as, low health literacy, meaning difficulty obtaining, processing, and understanding basic health information and appropriate services, poses an additional barrier (Sentell and Braun 2012; US Department of Health and Human Services 2000). Indeed, low health literacy correlates with poorer health (Sentell and Braun 2012). Yvette Flores proposes that "providers' lack of cultural attunement to the health beliefs of clients or patients, as well as a lack of culturally relevant services," also accounts for low utilization rates by Latino/as (2013, 3). Similarly, Rastogi and collaborators (2012) find that Latino/as in the US may avoid seeking care because of concerns about cultural misunderstandings and confronting racism. Indeed, mental health practitioners evaluate bilingual patients whose first language is Spanish differently when the interaction takes place in English than in Spanish (American Psychiatric Association 2017). In what Martínez (2011) terms the *linguistic gradient,* language ability correlates with the likelihood of receiving mental health care. For example, in one study, 43 percent of Latino/as who spoke English only sought and received mental health care, whereas 35 percent of bilingual Latino/as and 8 percent of those with limited English proficiency did so (Martínez 2011; Sentell et al. 2007). These findings serve to underscore the urgency of research on the health impacts that minority-language-speakers face.

Numerous studies in public health and epidemiology have provided substantial support for the role of culture in language during medical interactions (Davis et al. 2007; Eamranond et al. 2009; Ingram et al. 2007; Joshu et al. 2007; McEwen et al. 2010). For example, multiple studies that measured the effects of *promotoras*—community health promoters who have backgrounds similar to those of the patients they work with—on farmworkers with diabetes found significant improvements in health outcomes (Davis et al. 2007; Ingram et al. 2007; Joshu et al. 2007; McEwen et al. 2010). Patients who receive guidance from *promotoras* were more likely to discuss their concerns, both emotional and physical, about their diabetes with family members, friends, and their physicians following these interactions (Ingram et al. 2007). They also had improved glycemic control, which generally improves the long-term outcomes for diabetic patients (Ingram et al. 2007). While these studies do not address transcultural communication specifically, the design of the intervention suggests that it is present.

Latino/a practitioners are crucial in addressing language and cultural barriers and in offering Latino/as transcultural communication. However, another disparity in Latino health is the underrepresentation of Latino/as among practitioners. Only 5 percent of medical school graduates are Latino/a, and only 2 percent of full-time employed physicians are Hispanic (Association of American Medical Colleges 2016). Similarly, only 5 percent of psychologists identify as Hispanic (Lin et al. 2015). There are almost 3,500 Latino/as for every Latino/a mental health care professional, but only 578 non-Latino whites for every non-Latino white mental health care professional (Y. Flores 2013, 10). Even as the Latino population increases, the number of Latino/a doctors shows no sign of doing so (De la Torre and Estrada 2015). As well, the statistics understate the problem in that not all doctors with Latino backgrounds can deliver services in Spanish, and they may also lack cultural competency. Even some who speak Spanish may have difficulty because they don't have a command of the appropriate register to interact with their patients. As De la Torre and Estrada note, it is crucial for "medical providers to be sensitive to regional dialects of Spanish as well as the use and knowledge of idiomatic expressions and cultural beliefs of diseases to convey information about certain health disorders" (2015, 133).

Addressing Cultural Barriers

The national standards for culturally and linguistically appropriate services (CLAS) are designed to address language and cultural issues that minorities face in health care (Office of Minority Health 2013). They offer guidance to health care organizations aimed "to advance health equity, improve quality, and help eliminate health care disparities by establishing a blueprint for health and health care organizations" (66). Of the fifteen standards, four are explicitly dedicated to communication and language assistance: offer free language assistance to patients with limited English proficiency, inform patients of these services (in their language and writing), ensure the competence of those providing language assistance, and provide easy-to-understand written materials.

The CLAS standards are an important contribution to raising awareness among health care providers. But because they do not provide specific contextualized examples, they leave practitioners to figure out, for instance, what it would look like to "respect the cultural beliefs of others" in a real interaction. They also focus purely on medically oriented interactions, even though social-oriented interactions promote a stronger doctor–patient relationship (Cordella 2004; Coupland 2000; Maynard and Hudak 2008; Mishler 1984; Ragan 2000). Social-oriented interactions are central to the normative cultural values among Latino/as that have become commonplace in the literature on Latino health (Añez et al. 2005; Cordella 2004; Erzinger 1991; G. Flores 2000). These values[3] include the following:

Simpatía: kindness, friendly/relaxed exchange over interpersonal conflict
Personalismo: friendliness and prioritizing of interpersonal over institutional relationships
Respeto: deferential behavior based on age, gender, social position of the interlocutor
Confianza: mutual trust where the interpersonal aspects of the relationship are prioritized

These values are generally stronger for first-generation Latino immigrants than for later generations (Añez et al. 2005). Relying on these constructs is important for recently migrated Latino/as because it helps build community and networks to connect to critical sources of support (finding employment, housing, etc.), which is crucial in addressing the challenges of migration and cultural differences. Research documents that when health care practitioners take these values into account, patient distress in seeking treatment and treatment effectiveness decreases (Añez et al. 2005).

While research on cultural constructs has advanced awareness of cultural competency in health care, this approach misses knowledge of how authentic

---

3. Latino/as are a highly diverse group; not all will share these values. Further, these values may be more prominent for more recently migrated groups than for more acculturated Latino/as (Antshel 2002).

exchanges with patients reveal the deployment of Latino values and cultural constructs. Linguistic research could help bridge this gap through studies on how practitioners interact with Latino/a patients using both professional and informal registers of Spanish and offering contextualized examples of communication that is culturally appropriate and adapted to local communities. To understand how cultural competency unfolds in medical interactions, we need more linguistic studies that investigate how discourse unfolds in successful interactions with Spanish speakers in the US. This is especially important in a context where the Spanish language is the minority and where its speakers have social and health disadvantages.

Interpreted-Mediated Communication in Latino Health Care

Linguistics research has begun to shed light on specific problems in medical interactions affecting Spanish speakers in the US (Angelelli 2004; Davidson 2000, 2001; Martínez 2008, 2010, 2011; Raymond 2014a, 2014b). For example, Martínez's (2008) study in a geographic context that is predominantly Spanish-speaking along the US–Mexico border, collected semistructured interviews with thirty-four Spanish-speaking participants and revealed that they perceived English as superior to Spanish. Martínez also found that providers did not offer medical brochures written in Spanish and that interpreters, therefore, could only offer information by translating it orally, which put patients who were not literate in English at a clear disadvantage. Interpreters were often nonprofessionals, and Martínez found that they often did not deliver the doctor's statements in a way that was accessible to patients.

Interpreter training promotes the idea that the ideal interpreter is invisible to the patient, responsible only for interpreting the linguistics aspects of the conversation and ensuring mutual comprehension. However, research shows that interpreters have social agency—a significant role in shaping the interaction. This is inevitable given linguistic and cultural differences between interlocutors and the fact that interpreters are social beings in an interaction (Angelelli 2004; Davidson 2000). The California Healthcare Interpreting Association (CHIA) standards recognize the agentic role of interpreters by explaining that in addition to their roles as message converters and message clarifiers, they are also (or should be) cultural clarifiers and patient advocates. They call on interpreters to go "beyond message clarification to include a range of actions that typically relate to an interpreter's ultimate purpose of facilitating communication between parties not sharing a common culture. Interpreters are alert to cultural words or concepts that might lead to misunderstanding and act to identify and assist the parties to clarify culturally-specific ideas" (CHIA Standards and Certification Committee 2002, 14). As patient advocates, interpreters are responsible for supporting patients and recognizing that they will have a stance in the interaction, including making ethical decisions.

Nonetheless, interpreting does not provide the optimal solution to language barriers and patient care. Davidson's (2000, 2001) study of cross-linguistic interpreting in northern California reveals that interpreters obstruct the doctor–patient interpersonal relationship by editing and deleting conversational offerings. Specifically, interpreters acted as co-diagnosticians through selective interpretation. They received scant on-the-job training in medical discourse processes, and requirements in terms of knowledge of medical terms were minimal. In a finding quite different from Davidson's, an ethnographic study of interpreters (Angelelli 2004) reveals that they had ample knowledge of health care and advanced linguistic abilities, including cultural competence, accommodating to patients' registers, and skilled three-way communication. Yet, the study brings to light numerous prescriptive language attitudes that would limit interpreters' value. Most were middle-class Latino/as, and they explicitly discriminated against the registers of working-class Latino/a patients. For example, an interpreter described "people who have formal education as easier to talk with and people with less education as more difficult" (Angelelli 2004, 110). Another interpreter said that she would speak in any register to accommodate a patient but that she always began with the highest register and adjusted downward, an approach unlikely to make patients feel comfortable. Similarly, the interpreter described this process in stigmatizing terms, describing her starting point as riding an "elegant horse" and comparing speaking with some patients to "crawling" (Angelelli 2004, 113). Unfortunately, the implicit bias evident in this description appears to be common and left uncritiqued. For example, the book's author did not critique the interpreter's condescending views but instead portrayed her as skillful. The description of Spanish varieties that working-class speakers use as being of low prestige is ideological and is evidence of patronizing views of them. In this way, social issues of class can hamper meaningful communication. Spanish-speaking practitioners can readily fall into the same traps in assuming that the patient speaks the same "at-home" variety of Spanish as the doctor.

At the same time, Martínez explains that the problem lies in the very framing of interpretation as "language assistance," saying that it "create[s] policies that merely scratch the surface of the current problem" and that instead "policy should also consider language acceptance" (2011, 72). Language acceptance entails sociolinguistic awareness of the varieties of Latino/as in the US, a descriptive view of and attitude toward language varieties, and the ability to accommodate to the variety of patients in order to not mark, even subconsciously, inferiority/superiority distinctions between varieties.

The need for doctors and interpreters who are culturally and (socio)linguistically effective in their consultations with Spanish-speaking Latino/a patients is evident. This book aims to provide analyses that will support such effectiveness.

Doctor–Patient Discourse and Culture

While numerous studies have illuminated research on the social and discursive aspects of doctor–patient interactions, most have dealt with consultations in English. Discourse analysis studies have been conducted on Australian English in an emergency department (Slade et al. 2008), US English in various types of institutions (Ainsworth-Vaughn 1998; Ferrara 1994; Frankel 1990; Labov and Fanshel 1977; Stivers 2007; Stivers and Heritage 2001; West 1984), and British English in multicultural contexts involving genetic counseling and primary care (Roberts and Sarangi 2005).

Studies on provider–patient discourse in Spanish are scarce and mostly done in Spanish-dominant contexts such as Uruguay (Delbene 2004), the Dominican Republic (Bloom 2014; Bloom-Pojar 2018), and Chile (Cordella 2007). Among these, Marissa Cordella's *The Dynamic Consultation: A Discourse Analytical Study of Doctor–Patient Communication* (2004) is a book-length discourse on studies of doctor–patient communication in Spanish. It is based on the interactions of twenty-two patients and four doctors in Santiago, Chile, at an outpatient clinic. The resulting analysis offers numerous insights about cultural constructs among Spanish speakers such as *simpatía* (friendliness) and *confianza* (mutual trust) as well as the distinct voices that doctors and patients assume. However, the patients she studies do not face the same structural inequalities that affect Mexicans in California, specifically because they are not minority-language-speakers. These contexts influence language use and the relationship between doctors and patients. For example, Cordella (2004) describes a single case where a patient's lower socioeconomic background made it difficult to have a real connection with a doctor. In my study, all the patients are of a lower socioeconomic background than the doctor. At the same time, in the US environment, Dr. Ortiz and most of his patients share a minority identity as Mexican immigrants, which gives them an instant connection based on shared minority status.

Article-length works on US Spanish in health care interactions include studies of how providers strategically use politeness and mitigation in motivational interviews (Flores-Ferrán 2010, 2012). Erzinger's (1991) examination of doctor–patient Spanish interactions focuses on the values and culture of Latino/as in health care with a particular focus on *respeto* and *simpatía*, showing that these concepts illuminate the power dynamics between doctor and patient during medical consultations. Because of the cultural rule of *respeto,* patients in her study do not interrupt their doctors, which can lead them to fail to obtain needed clarifications. Erzinger also found that a provider who did not follow the rules of *respeto* and *simpatía* experienced conflicts with patients.

To date, practitioners cannot consult a systematic, comprehensive, detailed account of how Spanish-speaking Latino/as in the US communicate their health concerns or how they might realize transcultural communication in a particular US context. This book examines interactions in which the doctor and patients use a minority language, at times in stigmatized varieties. The repercussions for the building of trust are distinct from those in monolingual contexts. The patients whose discourse I studied are vulnerable because of their minoritized status, structural inequalities, and disproportionate health risks. Therefore, when a doctor aligns with these patients, solidarity is powerful. Further, this book considers the lexical and grammatical role of language in a social context: the context is bilingual, Spanish is the minority language, and health care is a context in which Latino/as are particularly vulnerable. For these reasons, a transcultural approach is most appropriate.

Approach to Linguistic Analysis

The study's theoretical approach, systemic functional linguistics (SFL), affords tools to analyze language from multiple levels of specification: genre, register, and interpersonal grammar (Halliday 1978; Halliday and Matthiessen 2004). It suits the book's core questions about transcultural communication and supports an analysis of how this discourse unfolds from a stratified system of language. Applying this theory to these cases explicitly reveals the cultural values and illustrates how this discourse unfolds at the level of language. SFL is appropriate because it allows for a holistic analysis of the language/stratified levels and its flexibility in allowing me to use other approaches (for example, I use sociolinguistics to analyze code-switching), including a critical lens, to discourse analysis. A number of recent health communication studies, primarily addressing English-language interactions, have employed SFL (De

TABLE 1. Register variable and language metafunctions

REGISTER	METAFUNCTION
tenor: relationship of interlocutors	**interpersonal:** negotiating personal relationships
field: social action taking place	**ideational:** constructing experience
mode: role of language	**textual:** organizing the text

Adapted from James R. Martin and David Rose, 2008, *Genre Relations: Mapping Culture* (London: Equinox).

Silva Joyce et al. 2015; Josephson et al. 2015; Matthiessen 2013; McDonald and Woodward-Kron 2016; Slade et al. 2008; Tebble 2008).

SFL is a social theory that describes language as a system of options that speakers use to make distinct meanings through their word and grammatical choices. Discourse, which consists of these language choices, is situated within social and cultural practices. Thus, it represents a contextualized understanding of language use. SFL views language as existing within a stratified system having three layers. The most abstract layer is culture, termed *genre* in this context. The specific situation in which language is used is the next layer, termed the *register*. The most concrete layer consists of language metafunctions: the *textual*, which is the flow and distribution of information; the *interpersonal*, which involves the negotiation of personal relationships; and the *ideational*, which concerns how we construct experience (Martin and White 2005, 1–7). All these metafunctions operate simultaneously and complement each other. Each of these metafunctions, in turn, functions with a variable of register: textual metafunction with mode, interpersonal metafunction with tenor (interlocutors), and ideational metafunction with field. Table 1 shows the relationships between the register variables and the language metafunctions and summarizes the concepts.

My analysis begins from the genre and proceeds to the register and then interpersonal metafunction. Figure 1 shows the overall relationship between genre, register, and language metafunctions. I focus specifically on the tenor strand from the different levels of language stratification to inspect the discourse between a doctor and his patients in depth. This stratified system of language affords analysis of the discourse from different levels of abstraction, where all metafunctions work together in every statement. A more holistic view of the language use in context thus emerges.

SFL affords the tools to discuss transcultural communication explicitly. It illuminates interpersonal meaning in the medical discourse, showing how both doctor and patient negotiate *simpatía, respeto, personalismo,* and *confianza.* These values are not independent of each other but instead can overlap.

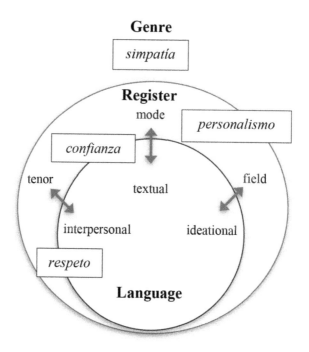

FIGURE 1. Language, genre, register, and cultural constructs

For instance, there is great overlap between *personalismo* and *simpatía*. This book proposes to offer specific, contextualized examples of these cultural constructs during real-time doctor–patient interactions. The examples throughout this book aim to raise awareness of how practitioners can deploy Latino values to make stronger connections between what is proposed in the literature and specific ways in which this is carried out. Based on the multilevel analysis, I discuss how *simpatía* takes place and how small talk leads to *personalismo* at the most abstract level during the course of the medical interview. I analyze more concrete levels in considering register, specifically, the role of participants. Here I focus on how *confianza* can take place through colloquialisms and bilingual practices; also, how interruptions and taboo language informs us of *respeto*. Finally, in analyzing the interpersonal language, the most concrete level, my data reveal politeness strategies that serve to show *respeto*.

Data: Study Participants and Interview Setting

The data for this study consist of twenty-three intake psychiatric interviews conducted in Visalia, California, two 45-minute follow-up interviews with Dr. Ortiz, who conducted the interviews, and numerous follow-up emails with him. These interviews were video recorded; however, I was not present during the recording. The recorded interviews were part of a larger study by researchers at the UC Davis Medical Center (Odor et al. 2011; Yellowlees et al. 2010; Yellowlees et al. 2011). All participants whose videos were collected for this study had given informed consent and agreed to allow their consultation sessions to be used for research and education purposes. I was given permission to conduct a secondary analysis and obtained institutional review board[4] approval from the University of California.

The interviews consist of an initial psychiatric assessment during which the doctor determines whether to recommend mental health care for the patients. They range from eighteen to forty-two minutes long. I transcribed each interview, which averaged 3,616 total words per consultation, with a total corpus of 83,169 words. Chapter 2 offers a more detailed analysis of the interview components.

Dr. Ortiz is a surgeon working at the intersection of health care, technology, and cultural inclusiveness. In our meetings and email discussions, I asked him questions about language and cultural issues affecting Latino/as in the US. He told me about his background, his strategies, and his approach to serving Spanish-speaking patients. The doctor differs culturally, linguistically, and socioeconomically from his patients. Dr. Ortiz was born in Mexico City and received his MD in Mexico. At the time of the interviews, he had been practicing medicine for more than thirty-three years, five of them in California. He is a middle-class, middle-aged man with a high level of education and a job that carries social status and power. He speaks English and several Spanish registers, including a prestige variety of Spanish and more colloquial registers, since he has been exposed to numerous language varieties given Mexico City's diversity. Before coming to California, he was a faculty member at a university and a physician in Mexico City, where he also worked with remote rural Mexican communities.

All twenty-three patients in this study were of Mexican descent. Most were born in rural areas of Mexico and moved to California's Central Valley as adults; four were born or raised in the US. Their Spanish includes features associated with rural Spanish and often has English-language influence. More than half the patients in this study were unemployed because of disability, retirement, or layoffs. The remainder performed manual labor as farmworkers, janitors, and construction workers. The patients range in education levels. Some who were raised in Mexico have only attended a few years of elementary school and are illiterate. A couple of the patients attended college, but

---

4. An institutional review board ensures the protection of the rights and welfare of human research subjects. The protocol number for this study is 247840-3.

none have bachelor's degrees. Appendix I contains a summary of the patients' backgrounds.

The sample size (twenty-three recorded consultations) allowed me to focus on fine-grained linguistic choices the speakers make to qualitatively describe their language in detail while also providing descriptive statistics revealing key linguistic patterns. Including one doctor as part of the study helps eliminate social variables. Had this study included more doctors, there would be additional variables that may impact patients' language choices, including doctors' gender, age, race, ethnicity, social status, personality, approach, technique, and experience. For example, if this study had involved several female and male doctors, it would have to account for gendered-based communication, shifting away from its language and culture focus.

Visalia, where Dr. Ortiz conducted the interviews, is about 200 miles north of Los Angeles. Agriculture drives the local economy. Half of Visalia's 133,010 people are Hispanic (US Census Bureau 2018). Latino/as are the majority group at 50.3 percent (most are of Mexican descent); non-Latino whites compose 40 percent of the population. Other groups include Asians, at 6 percent, and African Americans, at 2 percent (US Census Bureau 2018).

Poverty and low education levels are issues of grave concern in the Central Valley. Of the overall population in Visalia, one-fifth live at poverty levels (US Census Bureau 2018). Only 5 percent have a bachelor's degree, and 31 percent have less than a high school education. These disadvantages affect Latino/as disproportionately: 28 percent of Latino/as live in poverty, whereas 10 percent of non-Latino whites do, and only 11 percent of Latino/as have a bachelor's degree, whereas 30 percent of non-Latino whites do (US Census Bureau 2017).

The Spanish language has an important place in the Central Valley. In Visalia, about one-third of the population speaks a language other than English in the home, predominantly Spanish. Grocery stores, restaurants (including sit-down and fast food), barbershops, tax services, cell phone repairs (etc.), provide customer service in Spanish, and many display signs indicating "se habla español." At parks and soccer fields, street vendors sell Mexican treats like fruit cups prepared with lemon and spicy/sweet sauce; corn on the cob prepared with Mexican mayonnaise, Mexican cheese, and hot sauce; and raspado ice with flavors like tamarind, rompope (Mexican eggnog), coconut, hibiscus, walnut, and pineapple. Food trucks also serve authentic Mexican fare, and any of these vendors, as well as those who sell produce off the main roads or highway, may speak Spanish only. Driving on the main freeway that passes through the Central Valley, one sees billboards in Spanish, and on the radio many Spanish-speaking DJs play only music in Spanish.

Like much of California's Central Valley, Visalia has a shortage of health care professionals (Yellowlees et al. 2010). This is typical of rural areas and may explain the more significant health disparities that Latino/as in rural areas experience compared with urban Latino/as. For instance, Latino/as who live in rural areas are less likely to know about mental health resources available to them than Latino/as living in urban areas (García et al. 2011).

Overview of the Book

This book examines doctor–patient interactions in Spanish spoken in rural California to illuminate how transcultural competency unfolds at the linguistic level. This work provides linguistic insights into how rural Mexican patients narrate their experiences in a medical context and how they negotiate aspects of the roles related to social expectations and power dynamics. The study shows that creating an interpersonal relationship with Mexican patients involves small talk, humor, self-disclosure, and the use of informal language (e.g., bilingual practices and colloquialisms). I argue that doctors need transcultural knowledge of patients' social, linguistic, and cultural backgrounds to form an interpersonal relationship with them, and that in this way they can gain patients' trust and empower them. By explicitly articulating the discourse strategies that doctors can use in communicating with Latino/a patients and empowering them, this book aims to provide insights for health care practitioners and those who train them, as well as policymakers.

By examining interactions in Spanish spoken in rural California, this project addresses a critical gap in discourse analysis research. Chapter 2, "Psychiatric Interviews as a Genre and Patients' Narratives," serves to further contextualize the book by describing the elements that compose the interviews. Genre theory, within the SFL approach, affords the analytic tools to present abstract levels of psychiatric interviews (i.e., the macrolanguage or overall picture). It discusses the genre of the interview in terms of cultural expectations and practice. This section of the book offers examples of *simpatía* as a transcultural strategy that the doctor employs to help patients narrate their social and health stories. Doctors who cannot speak the language their patients speak may fail to obtain their health narratives. By documenting what occurs when a doctor elicits such narratives using techniques based on transcultural knowledge, I hope to support the gathering of such narratives in Spanish among practitioners, a crucial step toward humane health care.

Chapter 3, "*Hacer Plática*: Small Talk Subgenres," employs genre theory to inspect a vital component of the interviews: small talk. The chapter discusses not only the transcultural content of small talk but also the specific linguistic forms it takes. Genre theory reveals that small talk is more than simplified social exchanges; it is a complex interpersonal activity that can take the form of diverse genres, including anecdotes, gossip, humor, compliments, and personal advice. This chapter describes the doctor's *personalismo* and trans-culturally appropriate strategies, which play a crucial role in completing the medically oriented task even though they are outwardly socially oriented and interpersonal.

Chapter 4, "Register of the Psychiatric Interview: Interlocutors, Power, and Solidarity," focuses on a more micro-level analysis of the interviews. It considers the social and power roles of each interlocutor in light of the register of the psychiatric interview. At the discourse level, ways of claiming power include interrupting the interlocutor, posing questions, and using jargon. This chapter presents the results of each of these factors (how many questions each party poses; how many interruptions take place, and how; and the role of jargon in the interaction). It illustrates how the doctor mitigates the power distance between himself and patients through interpersonal communication and the creating of *confianza* (trust), a key cultural construct in psychiatric care. Interpersonal communication involves adapting to patients' registers, including using colloquialisms. It also reveals how the doctor maintains his more powerful role in the interaction by changing topics and interrupting patients. This chapter also points to sections in the interview where both doctor and patients show *respeto*.

Chapter 5, "Translanguaging in Health Care Interactions," offers insights into how *confianza* can be realized through *translanguaging,* which applied linguist Ofelia García influentially refers to as "multiple discursive practices in which bilinguals engage in order to make sense of their bilingual worlds" (2009, 45) The doctor aims to adapt the interview to the patient's language variety by translanguaging with several bilingual patients. This chapter describes how bilingual patients use their full linguistic repertoire beyond Spanish during the interview; for instance, they use English for medical terms. The doctor nourishes their translanguaging practices and further creates space for it when he uses English to clarify information. By engaging in translanguaging the doctor also demonstrates that he understands the complex and rich bicultural situation of bilingual patients and displays affective involvement as well as in-group knowledge. This chapter offers multiple examples of showing *confianza*. It provides unique ways by which interpersonal interactions empower patients to interact as fellow social beings, instead of solely as doctor and patient.

To explore interpersonal language choices in more detail, chapter 6, "Expressing Verbal Modality and Other Politeness Strategies in Psychiatric Interviews," focuses on various politeness strategies that doctors and patients use. Beyond the social power distance that exists between doctors and patients across cultures, for Latino/as there is an additional layer of social distance that comes with the cultural value of *respeto*. This chapter brings to light specific examples of *respeto* beyond using polite pronouns. Patients use politeness strategies such as modality at particular moments of psychiatric interviews, for instance, when discussing their symptoms and conditions to deliver their information carefully and to recognize the doctor's elevated social status. The doctor also strategically uses them when he asks sensitive questions to displace responsibility from the patients and show them *respeto*.

Chapter 7, "Conclusions: Spanish and Transcultural Discourse in Health, Teaching, and Research," reflects on the findings presented in earlier chapters using a sociocultural perspective of language to shed light on how transcultural strategies are explicitly realized. The doctor's interactions with the patients in this study provide numerous examples of transcultural communication that are adapted to the local community. These authentic exchanges between doctor and patients reveal the deployment of Latino values and cultural constructs and show how the doctor interacts with Latino/a patients in linguistically and culturally sensitive ways. The chapter draws on findings articulated in previous chapters to suggest practical implications of this research for health professionals.

Transcultural competence has become a particular focus for language researchers since the publication of the Modern Language Association's 2007 report *Foreign Languages and Higher Education: New Structures for a Changed World*. The report stresses the importance of a deep understanding of transcultural competence across multiple cultures, situations, and contexts (Geisler et al. 2007). Students commonly enroll in Spanish classes because they hope to use the language in their future profession (Carreira and Kagan 2011). This is true of both second-language and heritage-speaker students. However, very little linguistics research has explored the use of Spanish by US-based professionals; as a result, teachers of Spanish have had little guidance on the actual characteristics of "professional Spanish," which is often assumed to be the generic, hyper-standard world Spanish found in textbooks. In many classrooms, heritage speakers are still told that the Spanish they learned at home is "incorrect." In others, they are told that their home Spanish is fine to use with their family but that they should not speak that way in professional contexts (Villa 2010). In most US university classrooms, code-switching between Spanish and English is frowned upon because of the belief that languages should not be mixed in formal communication.

Meanwhile, second-language learners of Spanish often reach advanced levels in the classroom without much awareness of the language variation that exists worldwide and within US communities. This research implies that all these approaches fail to prepare students for many real-world professional contexts in which Spanish is used. Yet, both informal registers of speaking and specialized use of the language (medical Spanish) are required to make an interpersonal connection with another speaker. Textbooks on medical Spanish have heavily focused on the latter; as a result, practitioners emerge with little knowledge about the informal registers or their translanguaging practices (Hardin 2012; Ortega and Prada 2020).

This book focuses on language that conveys familiarity, meaning informal registers, because these interpersonal interactions are often overlooked in medical Spanish textbooks, which tend to emphasize formal language. One of the problems with the current approach in the medical textbooks is that they lack discussion of practical issues that medical professionals encounter, including knowledge about people's social values and how people discuss issues in colloquial or regional ways use such as regionalisms, colloquialisms, implicatures (Hardin 2012).

The research questions that the following chapters examine move from the basic conditions that provide context for the doctor's interviews to in-depth analysis of the components that impact the success of doctor–patient interactions in this context. By using multiple levels of linguistic analysis, I seek to provide a holistic representation of patient voices and health narratives. The data offer numerous examples of Dr. Ortiz's success in communicating with patients because of his knowledge of the language, culture, values, practices, and language socialization of patients, all of which are expressed and revealed within the discourse. I also provide linguistic insights concerning rural varieties of Spanish in the US, for example, in my analysis of how patients narrate their experiences in a medical context and how the doctor and his patients make small talk. This evidence is informative for protocols of medical professionals working with Spanish-speaking communities in the US.

This book speaks both to scholars working in humanities-oriented approaches to health, language, and culture, and to health and education practitioners and policymakers seeking to improve communication in health care. Each chapter concludes with a list of insights for medical interpreters and practitioners. Explicit awareness of language is especially crucial in the medical field, where resources are limited and practitioners are rushed continuously for time. Making brief interactions with patients meaningful and making purposeful word choices is a step toward creating more patient-centered care that values, recognizes, and strives to create the appropriate space for the language and culture of minority groups. As the number of Latino/as in the US continues to grow, it is vital that practitioners consider the culture of the patient, and evidencing such consideration through language can improve the care they provide.

Insights for Medical Practitioners and Interpreters

- Practitioners can gain their patients' trust through accurate translations of medical terminology, transcultural competency, and interpersonal interactions. Several cultural constructs that Latino/as consider essential to building relationships are based on interpersonal communication, including *simpatía, respeto, personalismo,* and *confianza. Confianza* (mutual trust) plays a crucial role in any medical interaction, as it makes it easier for patients to discuss their concerns and, in turn, obtain good-quality health care. Becoming more aware of interpersonal language is an essential step in proving transculturally competent care and making stronger connections with Spanish-speaking Latino/as.

- Language varieties can be stigmatized, and can create implicit biases. This stigma reflects class distinctions rather than intrinsic value, comprehensibility, or aesthetic features. It is crucial that practitioners and interpreters practice language acceptance (Martínez 2011). Practitioners should not mark, even subconsciously, inferiority/superiority distinctions between varieties. They should be aware of (though not necessarily conversant in) the varieties of Latinos in the US, hold a descriptive view of and attitude toward language varieties, and make strides to adapt conversation to patients' language variety.

CHAPTER 2

Psychiatric Interviews as a Genre and Patients' Narratives

THIS CHAPTER DRAWS on genre analysis in linguistics to approach Dr. Ortiz's psychiatric interviews. Genre analysis is useful in medical contexts because it allows us to reflect on and appreciate how language interactions occur in urgent situations (Slade et al. 2008). In the psychiatric interview genre, patients reveal intimate details about themselves through stories and details that become crucial when the doctor makes recommendations. Compared with other kinds of medical interviews, psychiatric interviews pose challenges to doctors and patients alike because of the delicate nature of the topics under discussion. To communicate the problems they experience, patients must tell stories and reveal deep-rooted issues to someone they are meeting for the first time. Genre analysis supports an explicit and detailed description of the language that both doctor and patients use as they negotiate the interviews and reveals the context of the culture, primarily through offering an abstract way to analyze the genres' components. In doing so, it draws attention to the culture of the local community. As linguist Suzanne Eggins (2004) asserts, genre analysis is a powerful step toward making explicit the cultural and social basis of language. This chapter reveals (1) genres and subgenres that are present in the psychiatric interview and their functions, (2) the types of genres patients draw upon when telling their stories, and (3) the transculturally informed types of discursive strategies the doctor employs. The chapter identifies how rural Mexican varieties influence how speakers interact with the genre of psychiatric interviews. It also reveals the transcultural discourse strategies that Dr. Ortiz uses to encourage patients to participate in this new genre. Research shows that fears that doctors in the US will misunderstand, judge, discriminate, or cause deportation prevent some Latino/a patients from seeking medical attention (Barr and Wanat 2005; Nieves-Ruiz 2010; Raymond-Flesch et al. 2014), making these transcultural strategies a critical public health measure in building trust among Latino communities. For instance, providers should work to strategically negotiate meaning in medical discourse in order to provide patients effective health care, creating a trustworthy environment when cultural barriers complicate this process.

Genre Theory

Genre theory within systemic functional linguistics (SFL) is "a staged, goal-oriented social process. Social because we participate in genres with other people, goal-oriented because we use genres to get things done, staged because it usually takes us a few steps to reach our goals" (Martin and Rose 2007, 8). Genres are rhetorical categories that depend on social structures and relate to one another intertextually. As Tardy points out, they "reflect and enforce existing structure[s] of power" (2011, 55). Thus, linguistics theories of genre (Labov and Waletzky 1997; Martin and Rose 2008) are well suited to reveal the language of psychiatric interviews explicitly and in a culturally situated context.

SFL understands genres as semiotic functions specific to the text. Genres have a social value in the culture and refer to the forms the language takes to obtain culturally appropriate objectives, that is, the general purpose of the interaction (Eggins 2004). Genre analysis shows us how interlocutors accomplish an interaction and allows us to inspect each component of the interaction. Each structural component serves a particular role in shaping the genre. Within these schematic structures, this study explores the types of subgenres that speakers engage in to make meaning. Subgenres occur within the overall genre and have a role just as important as that of the overall genre.

I assigned subgenres to the interviews deductively, reading them to find recurrent subgenres in the interviews. Some of the subgenres I identified have not appeared in the literature because they are specific to medical interviews and have not been studied using genre analysis. In this process, I identified both form and function; this chapter focuses on the functional component of seven interviews. Throughout the analysis, I highlight how discursive patterns reveal how transcultural communication can occur among local community speakers in the Central Valley and precisely how the doctor displays *simpatía*. The examples that appear here illustrate a representative range of patient situations (both medical and social) and the distinct ways that patients construct their stories. As the analysis below shows, Dr. Ortiz co-creates some of the stories with the patients through communication that is both linguistically and culturally concordant. This chapter also identifies interpersonal strategies that demonstrate the doctor's transcultural knowledge of his patients.

The Psychiatric Interview: Medical Perspectives

Daniel Carlat (2012), who teaches psychiatry at Tufts University, authored *The Psychiatric Interview*, an influential manual that medical students in psychiatry have been using for over two decades. The textbook instructs practitioners to complete the following tasks: build a therapeutic alliance (opening phase), obtain the psychiatric database and/or interview for diagnosis (body of interview), and negotiate a treatment plan with the patient (closing phase). The function of the opening phase is to meet patients and learn about them. During the body of the interview, the interviewer collects a history of present illness, family history of these disorders, sociodevelopmental history, and the patient's medical history and determines whether the patient meets the criteria for a specific condition. Finally, in the closing phase, the interviewer is supposed to discuss an appropriate assessment and negotiate a treatment plan with the patient.

From a linguistics point of view, the three phases are broad. For the current study, the fact that the presumed patient speaks English as a first language limits the usefulness of this conventional understanding for analyzing Dr. Ortiz's interviews. Further, these approaches give little attention to patients' perspectives in formulating their advice. To address this gap, the present chapter takes a closer look at the generic components of the psychiatric interview, as Dr. Ortiz practiced it. This chapter illustrates the role of language used by both Dr. Ortiz and his patients, highlighting how patients tell their health stories and specific examples in which the doctor mediates culturally diverse situations.

This analysis is designed to counter another problem with instructional texts: the minimal attention they pay to the interpersonal stages of psychiatric interviews. Even when advice acknowledges that these stages are key for patient comfort and trust, and that these elements affect clinical outcomes, the advice given on interpersonal interactions is often general and may not apply to minority groups. This chapter reinforces the importance of the interpersonal and socially oriented sections of the interview, treating both as formal schematic components of the psychiatric interview. The next section demonstrates the power of genre analysis for this chapter's aims.

The Genre of Psychiatric Interviews

Genre analysis of Dr. Ortiz's psychiatric interviews reveals that the schematic structure of the interviews largely conforms to forms he completes and uses as a guide. The first is a history form based on the *Diagnostic and Statistical Manual of Mental Disorders: DSM-IV* (First et al. 1997) that includes information on psychiatric and medical history, a mental status examination, substance abuse, medication, and social and developmental history. The other form is a Spanish version of the Mini-International Neuropsychiatric Interview that he uses to screen for psychiatric disorders (Sheehan et al. 1998). The following are the stages that conform to the topics on the forms. A caret "∧" indicates sequence:

> Greeting ∧ small talk [recurrent[1]] ∧ interview procedure ∧ demographic data ∧ history of present illness ∧ substance abuse and past medical history ∧ social and developmental history ∧ screening of psychiatric disorders ∧ conclusion

Within the generic components of the psychiatric interviews, certain subgenres recurred: instructions, anecdotes, short answers, personal exchanges, narratives, and recounts. Table 2 shows the connections between the generic components and the subgenres.

The sections below provide examples of the genres and subgenres from the interviews. A complete transcription of one of the interviews is available in appendix II.

Greeting

Each interview begins with a greeting where a patient and the doctor introduce themselves. It typically involves a handshake, smiles, saying names, and "*mucho gusto*"—"pleased to meet you." Dr. Ortiz always goes into the waiting room to greet his patients; thus, this portion of the interview begins there. During my interview with Dr. Ortiz, he explained to me that allowing office staff to bring his patients back creates more distance. This way, the rest of the interview takes place in a room unfamiliar to the patient, but not with a completely unfamiliar person. Research shows that greetings are crucial for

---

1. Small talk is a recurrent generic component that can occur multiple times throughout an interview but is more common toward the beginning.

TABLE 2. Summary of generic components of psychiatric interviews, subgenres, and function

GENERIC COMPONENTS	SUBGENRES	FUNCTION
Greeting	personal exchange	introduce each other
Small talk	anecdote, recount, personal exchange	establish interpersonal relationship, warm-up
Interview procedure	instructions	educate the patient
Demographic information	short response, personal exchange	collect basic patient information, warm-up, establish interpersonal relationship
History of present illness	recount, narrative, personal exchange	collect description of symptoms
Substance abuse, past medical history	short response, personal exchange	collect past medical history
Sociodevelopmental history	narrative, personal exchange	collect patients' stories to understand their contexts
Screening for psychiatric disorders	instructions, short response, personal exchange	determine follow-up treatment
Conclusion	personal exchange	conclude the consultation

building an alliance between patients and doctors, and Dr. Ortiz shows an intuitive understanding of this (Carlat 2012). He also demonstrates knowledge of *simpatía,* since by walking with the patient to the consultation room, he is signaling to them that he will take extra steps to make them feel welcomed.

Small Talk

In virtually all the interviews, small talk follows or precedes the greeting. Small talk refers to any type of interpersonal chatting that is not specifically related to diagnosis and can occur at any point in the interview. Small talk is critical for setting a comfortable environment for the patient from the beginning of the interview and for building trust between patient and doctor, particularly in a sensitive setting like the psychiatric interview (Coupland 2000; Ragan 2000; Stivers and Heritage 2001). Because the next chapter focuses on small talk, I only note its presence and importance here.

Explanation of Interview Procedure

After greetings and making small talk, Dr. Ortiz explains the procedure of the interview and the types of questions the patient can expect. I label the subgenre that characterizes this part of the interview *Instructions*. Instructions consist of an optional orientation, a direction, and an interpretation. The doctor explains that he will ask questions similar to those that a general medical provider asks but that they will focus on psychological problems. This procedural explanation helps familiarize the patient with the genre of the interview. For patients with little experience with medical consultations, it is particularly important. The explanation of the procedure demonstrates the doctor's role as the expert, showing his wealth of experience performing such interviews and assessments as he shares this knowledge with patients.

Language shifts significantly between the greeting and small talk phase and the procedural explanation. Whereas the greeting and small talk have *interpersonal meaning*, which the doctor uses to form a relationship with the patient, in describing psychiatric interviews the doctor's language has *ideational meaning*, which refers to how experiences are constructed (Martin and White 2005). In this case, the experience refers to engaging a patient in a psychiatric interview. The doctor offers instructions to prepare patients for the interview, as illustrated in a consultation with a woman in her late forties:

1) Interview procedure

Orientation

Dr. Ortiz: *Mire, lo que vamos a hacer es esto:*
             Look, what we are going to do is this:

Direction 1

Dr. Ortiz: *Primero le voy a hacer nada más esta hoja*
             First I am going to have you do this sheet

Interpretation 1

Dr. Ortiz: *que es como una consulta como la que le da John pero con más*
             énfasis en sus problemas psicológicos
             it's like a consultation like the one John gives you but with more
             emphasis on your psychological problems

Direction 2

Dr. Ortiz: *y después le voy a hacer unas preguntas*
             and then I am going to ask you some questions

Interpretation 2

Dr. Ortiz: *y a estas preguntas, me tiene que decir sí o no nada más.*
             to these questions, you just have to just answer yes or no.

The orientation, "*Mire, lo que vamos a hacer es esto,*" functions to prepare the patient for the instructions. The doctor's first direction indicates the history form. The doctor interprets this direction by drawing on his previous knowledge of the patient and making a connection between the current form and the forms that her general practitioner has completed, pointing out a key difference in the questions he will pose. The next direction is that the patient will answer certain questions, to which she should respond with a simple "yes/no" answer (interpretation). The doctor-interpretations are interpersonal parts of these instructions that the face-to-face nature of the interview influences. While the directions are medically oriented, the interpretations are more socially oriented. Perhaps in written "instructions," interpretations would be absent; however, in the face-to-face context of the psychiatric interview, they are important components because they influence how the interlocutors establish their interpersonal relationship. Through these interpretations, the doctor lets the patient know that he speaks in her register and therefore aligns with her.

Demographic Information

The demographic information the doctor seeks includes date of birth, place of birth, employment, social benefits, hobbies, occupation, religious affiliation, marital status, and length of residence in the US. The patients provide brief answers, and, in many cases, either interlocutor adds personal exchanges, which are socially oriented instead of task-oriented. In the following example, the patient, Trinidad, a woman in her mid-sixties (#11), demonstrates a desire for informal interactions:

2) Demographic information

Short Response

Dr. Ortiz: ¿*Usted cuándo nació Trinidad?*
When were you (formal) born Trinidad?

Trinidad: *Uuh, yo nací [date] del 44. Así es de que ya 65 años oiga.*
Oh wow, I was born on [date], 1944. So, yes, I'm already 65 years old, sir.

Personal Exchange

Dr. Ortiz: *Ándele.*
There you (formal) go.

Trinidad: *Ya me pesan los años, ya, ya, ya, no crea.*
The years are taking a toll on me.

The doctor does not specifically ask her for her age, but the patient offers this information anyway, giving the communication a more conversational style as opposed to a short and simple answer, which the patient may perceive as rude. The doctor displays *simpatía* by answering with "*ándele*," a colloquialism, to acknowledge the additional information. The patient's remark about the years taking a toll expresses personal feelings about her age and reminds the doctor that she has a daughter (not present), making the interview more conversational and connecting on a more interpersonal level. Through her personal exchange, the patient uses a subgenre she is familiar with to complete a less-familiar task of answering medical interview questions; the patient is negotiating genre conventions. At the same time, the patient claims power by taking control of the conversation and initiating this informal topic in a setting where usually the doctor controls the agenda and the topic of conversation through his questions (Ainsworth-Vaughn 1998).

History of Present Illness

From the doctor's point of view, learning the history of present illness is the most crucial part of the psychiatric interview. Some doctors emphasize the most recent experiences of the patient; others believe in collecting the entire history. During this stage, Dr. Ortiz collects a wealth of information from patients' histories (although the amount of scaffolding he does varies across patients). The topics of this subgenre include comorbid conditions, legal concerns, relationships and family problems, and financial worries. Recounts and narrative responses are common during the history of present illness.

His interaction with Roberto (a male patient in his forties, #8), is typical, although some patients provide a more elaborate narrative in response to similar questions:

3) History of present illness as a recount
Dr. Ortiz: *Entonces, ¿por qué lo mandó [doctor's name] para acá?*
              Well then, why did [doctor's name] send you here?
Orientation
Roberto: *Ah, porque dice que . . . que creo que tengo la enfermedad
              mentalmente.*
              Oh, because he says that . . . I believe I have a mental illness.
Dr. Ortiz: *Uh-huh.*
Record of Events
Roberto: *Siempre parece que me estoy ahogando.*
              I always feel like I'm drowning.

Dr. Ortiz: *Uh-huh.*

Record of Events

Roberto: *No siempre, cuando hay problemas o algo, siento que me falta aire.*
Not always, when there are problems or something, I feel out of breath.

Dr. Ortiz: *Uh-huh.*

Reorientation

Roberto: *Por eso me dijo.*
That's why he told me.

Dr. Ortiz consistently uses the referring doctor's name in these inquiries and establishes his connection to someone the patient knows and perhaps trusts. However, he does not reference any information the general practitioner has given him. The patient uses a recount to summarize his main concern ("mental illness") and explain his symptoms of breathlessness, which are the record of events. The patient delivers this information through negotiation with the doctor, who encourages him to explain his symptoms further. In this example, we note that the doctor uses the continuer discourse marker *uh-huh* to acknowledge the information and convey his attentiveness and pauses to allow the patient to construct the recount. The pause functions as a cue that the patient should continue. My findings resemble those of Cordella (2004), who also finds that continuer discourse markers encourage patients to continue to speak and let them know that they are being heard. This patient continues to elaborate on his symptoms, completing the reorientation constituent of the subgenre. The co-construction in which the doctor participates is passive in the sense that Dr. Ortiz does not ask specific questions to help this patient elaborate on his stories.

Another interaction, with Ramón (a male patient in his thirties, #13), leads to a more elaborate story:

4) History of present illness as a short response

Short Responses

Dr. Ortiz: *¿Por qué te ve* [doctor's name] *en la clínica?*
Why does [doctor's name] see you at the clinic?

Ramón: *Oh, porque tengo* high blood pressure *de mi mente y el hígado*
Oh, because I have high blood pressure because of my mind and the liver.

Dr. Ortiz: *¿El hígado qué tiene?*
What's going on with the liver?

Ramón: *'toy poquito malo del hígado [ininteligible], me dio medicina.*
I am a little ill because of the liver [unintelligible], he gave me medicine.

Dr. Ortiz: *Pero no tienes cirrosis.*
But you don't have cirrhosis.
Ramón: *No. Aquí también ando malo del . . .*
No. Right here too [points to his throat] I am ill because of
Dr. Ortiz: *¿Tiroides?*
Thyroid?
Ramón: [nods]
Dr. Ortiz: *Y de la mente, ¿qué tienes?*
And with the mind? What's going on?
Ramón: *A veces hablo cosas que no debo hablar. Se me va la mente así* [points away from himself].
Sometimes I say stuff that I shouldn't say. My mind drifts off like this.

When the doctor asks Ramón why his general practitioner sees him, the patient reveals issues with high blood pressure, his liver, thyroid, and "the mind." The doctor doesn't inquire immediately about the mental issues but instead probes further into the patient's liver problems, which helps the provider understand the patient's medical history thoroughly and lead to the patient's mental health problems more sensitively. After taking notes on his medical history, the doctor asks about the patient's mental health history, which triggers the patient to narrate his brain surgery experience:

5) History of present illness as a narrative

Abstract
Ramón: *Cuando 'taba chiquillo, me caí asina. Me tuvieron que hacer* surgery, brain surgery.
When I was little, I fell down. They had to operate on me, brain surgery.

Orientation
Dr. Ortiz: *¿Te hicieron* brain surgery?
They did brain surgery on you?
Ramón: *Sí, allá en Texas.*
Yes, over there in Texas.

Complication
Ramón: *Me caí de la troca de mi apá. Caí asina.*
I fall down from my dad's truck. I fall down like this.
Dr. Ortiz: *¿Cuántos años tenías?*
How old were you?

Ramón: *Unos cinco años. Por andar jugando en los monkey bars, me caí*
           asina. Estaba en una coma. No supe nada más. Miré la luz.
           I was about five years old. Because of playing on the monkey
           bars, I fell down like this. I was in a coma. I didn't know any-
           thing else. I saw the light.

Dr. Ortiz: *¿Cuánto tiempo estuviste en coma?*
           How long were you in a coma?

Ramón: *Seis horas.*
           Six hours.

Dr. Ortiz: *Seis horas.*
           Six hours.

Ramón: *Seis horas.*
           Six hours.

Dr. Ortiz: *¿Y te hicieron* brain surgery? *Y qué tenías ¿sangre?*
           And they did brain surgery on you? And what was going on,
           bleeding?

Ramón: *Me, me*
           They, they [gestures at his head making a circle] [hesitates]

Dr. Ortiz: [interrupts] *¿Te rompiste el cráneo?*
           Did you break your skull?

Ramón: *Sí.*
           Yes.

Evaluation

Ramón: *Ya mero me moría.*
           I almost died.

Resolution

Ramón: *Nomás que me salvaron.*
           But they saved me.

Ramón uses a narrative structure to tell his story, beginning with a summary
or abstract (the accident and brain surgery), an orientation (geography, Texas),
the main complication (falling off monkey bars, going into a coma, and getting
brain surgery), then an evaluation (that he almost died), and a resolution (the
doctors saved him). Dr. Ortiz participates actively in co-constructing the narrative by asking the patient specific questions (sometimes by interrupting), asking
how old the patient was at the time, how long he was in a coma, the problems
the fall had caused, and whether the surgery involved breaking bones.

Patients tend to describe their symptoms using descriptive terms like
desesperada/o (anxious), *triste* (sad), and *nerviosa/o* (nervous). When inquir-

ing further, the doctor strategically uses the patient's term, such as in this interaction with Josefina (a female patient in her late forties, #1) who says she feels sadness "*tristeza*":

6) History of present illness as a recount

Orientation

Dr. Ortiz: *¿Cómo es esa tristeza?*
What is that sadness like?

Josefina: *Pues una tristeza a veces que me dan ganas de llorar y hay veces que—*
Well sadness that sometimes makes me want to cry and sometimes—

Dr. Ortiz: *¿Llora fácil?*
Do you cry easily?

Record of Events

Josefina: *Sí, hasta eso que sí. Y hay veces que no tengo tristeza así. Y hay veces que pasa una cosa y no me da susto. Hasta otro día es cuando me agarran los nervios.*
Yes, even that I do. And there are times when I'm not sad like that. And there are times that something happens, and I get *susto*. The following day is when I get *nervios*.

Dr. Ortiz: *¿Cuándo se pone triste, cómo está su apetito?*
When you're sad, how is your appetite?

Josefina: *Pues no me da hambre.*
Well, I do not get hungry.

Dr. Ortiz: *¿Y cómo duerme?*
And how is your sleep?

Josefina: *Pues duermo mucho. Yo, si yo estoy dormida es mejor para mí porque no siento mis enfermedades.*
Well I sleep a lot. If I am asleep it is better for me because that way I don't feel my illnesses.

Dr. Ortiz: *Bien, y esta tristeza que le da a usted, ¿siente que es así como que sube y baja?*
Alright, and that sadness that you feel, do you feel like it goes up and down?

Reorientation

Josefina: *Sí.*
Yes.

Here the doctor interrupts the patient when she mentions crying to ask whether she cries easily. The doctor scaffolds the interaction by guiding the patient to voice her thoughts and feelings through his specific questions. Josefina's final "*Sí*" functions as a reorientation because it concludes that her sadness fluctuates. Recounts are not surprising during this portion of the interview because patients discuss problems they are currently struggling with and that have not been solved. Therefore, their medical issues lack a resolution (in terms of the generic structure), at least during the moment of the interview.

The range of scaffolding the doctor provides to help patients construct their medical histories varies. Some patients offer detailed histories with important details. In other cases, patients offer insufficient information (such as Josefina), and the doctor asks numerous questions to help them detail their symptoms. In this way, Dr. Ortiz assumes a more active role and co-constructs patients' experiences.

In talking with Amalia (a female patient in her mid-seventies, #20), Dr. Ortiz provides less guidance, but he demonstrates engagement in her story by nodding and taking notes. This patient gives a long answer that takes on a narrative structure. To analyze Amalia's narrative, I draw on Labov and Waletzky's (1997) description of narratives of personal experience as well as the "stages" approach that Martin and Rose (2008) propose, as in example 7:

7) History of present illness as a narrative

Abstract

Amalia: *Mire, me da mucha depresión por mi marido porque él no me apoya para nada.*
Look, I get depressed a lot because of my husband because he doesn't support me at all.

Orientation

setting: *Para él yo no valgo, yo estoy loca, yo nomás quiero cosas buenas*
To him I'm worthless, I'm crazy, I just want nice things

reaction: *y no es verdad que quiero cosas buenas*
and it's not true that I want nice things

setting 2: *porque si yo—Ahorita ya estamos retirados, ya no puedo trabajar.*
because if I—Right now we're retired, I can't work anymore.

Complication

problem 1: *Desde que me salió un tumor tan grande y luego enseguida me dio el* stroke, *me dio un ataque al corazón, pues ya definitivamente.*
Ever since I got a very big tumor, and then right after I had a stroke, I had a heart attack, well that's definitely it [with working].

problem 2:	*Y dice, tú nomás quieres puras cosas buenas, yo no puedo dártelas.*
	And he says, you just want nice things, I can't give them to you.
reaction:	*Le digo, nunca me las has dado. Sí me gusta lo bueno. No lo niego, pero hasta donde puedo, hasta donde alcanzo.*
	I tell him, you've never given them to me. Yes, I do like nice stuff. I won't deny it, but only what I can get, what I can afford.
reflection:	*Y es mucho sufrir.*
	And it's a lot of suffering.
problem 3:	*Tenemos separados ya de cuarto, de todo. Vivimos juntos, pero—pero ya no somos esposos. Tenemos trece años.*
	We have separated, [separate] rooms, everything. We live together but—but we're not husband and wife anymore. We've been like this for thirteen years.

Evaluation

evaluation:	*Entonces yo tengo muchas cosas que a veces—que me paro en la puerta de su cuarto. A veces tengo tanto miedo en mi cuarto, que alguien habló, ayy, escucho algo. Me voy con mi pillow en la mano, le digo, "¿me dejas quedarme contigo?"*
	So there are many things that sometimes—that I'll stand in front of his door. Sometimes I'm so scared in my room, like someone spoke, ohh, I hear something. With a pillow in my hand, I ask him, "can I stay the night with you?"
problem:	*No. [Se encoge de hombros y cruza brazos].*
	No. [She shrugs her shoulders and crosses her arms].
reaction:	*Me regreso y me pongo a llorar mucho.*
	I return [to my room] and I start crying a lot.
reflection:	*porque digo, "¿por qué yo le ando rogando?"*
	Because I tell myself, "why am I begging him?"

Resolution

reflection 1:	*No tengo por qué hacer eso.*
	I don't have to do that.
solution:	*Y ya me digo, "Dios mío, dame fuerzas."*
	And I tell myself, "My lord, give me strength."
reflection 2:	*Yo no tengo porque rogarle.*
	I don't have to beg him.

At the start of her narrative, Amalia provides an "abstract" (summary) of her story, saying she has depression because her husband doesn't support her at all. This is the main problem that she presents in her narrative and returns to at the end of her story. Within the orientation, the setting, a phase that offers a deeper level of analysis, introduces us to the context of the narrative: Amalia's health issues and marriage. At the end of her narrative, we see how her health complications tie into her central theme: the broken relationship with her husband.

In the second phase, the orientation, Amalia provides additional details to sketch the setting. She explains how she perceives her husband's feelings toward her, the problems that they are facing, and their retired status, which suggests that they have little money.

Amalia presents several complications in her narrative, including multiple health issues and problems in her relationship with her husband. She says that her husband complains that she wants things that they can't afford, but she disagrees. Her health problems and financial status magnify the intensity of her situation. Amalia reflects on these problems, saying that "*es mucho sufrir.*" Then she describes separate bedrooms and alludes to what appears to be a cessation of intimacy in her marriage. These complications build some suspense in this narrative. For example, the health issues are significant, but in this section, they are introduced to build suspense about her relationship with her husband and serve to further portray herself as a victim in her situation.

In the evaluation, Amalia presents her problems and offers a specific example to illustrate what she is going through, describing her husband's rejection when she desires his company. The patient describes her reaction, tears, and asking herself why she is "begging."

The final generic structure that the patient includes (and one that is oblig- atory for this story to be considered a narrative) is a resolution, asking her God for strength. This resolution also functions as a coda since it brings per- spective back to the present moment. At the grammatical level, we note that the patient uses the present tense "*Yo no tengo porque rogarle*" indicating her current standing.

In sum, the types of questions the doctor asks during the history of present illness elicit narrative responses and recounts. The doctor helps co-construct these stories by being an active or passive participant.

Sociodevelopmental History

Sociodevelopmental questions are particularly important in psychiatric inter- views since they give clinicians a more holistic view of the patient. As Carlat notes in his textbook, "The social history is useful in two closely related ways:

(a) it allows you to get to know the patient as a *person* rather than as a *diagnosis,* and (b) you can approach the diagnosis of a personality disorder through the social history" (2012, 113). At one time, Freudian influence dictated that practitioners spend hours probing to complete this portion of their interviews.

The sociodevelopmental history has an entirely different configuration from the history of present illness. This has consequences for how the doctor exercises his transcultural competence. In collecting the sociodevelopmental history, the doctor begins by probing into some of the patient's childhood history, which sometimes means eliciting repetition, as some patients have already offered this information earlier in the interview. Like the history of present illness, the sociodevelopmental history elicits a narrative response, but patients use recounts as well.

When initiating the sociodevelopmental history phase, the doctor asks questions that he tailors to each patient, such as referencing the patient's birthplace, which he learned from the demographic information phase, in asking about their childhood. In terms of genre, as with the histories of the present condition phases, patients choose narratives more than any other genre to describe their presenting problem. In numerous instances, the doctor has an active role in co-construing these narratives. Even talkative patients often find this phase emotionally difficult, such as Norma (a female patient in her mid-forties, #12):

8) Sociodevelopmental history as a narrative

Dr. Ortiz: *¿Y cómo fue su niñez en Jalisco?*
And how was childhood in Jalisco?

Orientation

Norma: *[Viéndose los pies] Pues a la vez—pues a la vez un niño yo pienso que a la mejor vive feliz, pero pues también embeces pasan muchas cosas que embeces no eres feliz, que embeces pues no sabes como puede ser la vida—[silencio].*
[Looking at her feet] Well at times—well at times a kid, I think that maybe they live happily but well sometimes some things also happen that sometimes you realize you are not happy, that sometimes well you don't know how life can be—[silence].

Dr. Ortiz: *¿Su mamá y su papá vivían en la casa?*
Did your mother and father live at home?

Complication 1

Norma: *No.*

Dr. Ortiz: *¿No? ¿No estaban con ustedes?*
No? They were not with you all?

Norma: *Mi papá no.*
          My father was not.
Dr. Ortiz: *¿Su papá no? ¿Su mamá sí?*
          Your father was not? Your mother was?

Evaluation 1

Norma: *[Se limpia una lágrima] Sí, mi mamá sí. Pobre, mi mamá—fuimos ocho—*
          [Wipes a tear] Yes, my mom, yes. My poor mom—there were eight of us—
Dr. Ortiz: *[Se levanta y sale de cuadro en busca de una toalla].*
          [Gets up and leaves the room to get a tissue].
Norma: *[Ve al suelo].*
          [Looks down].
Dr. Ortiz: *[Entra al cuarto]. Traje un súper Kleenex porque no hay dos. ¿Son ocho hermanos?*
          [Enters the room]. I brought a super Kleenex because there weren't two. There are eight siblings?
Norma: *Ocho conmigo. Somos—son siete hermanos y yo, somos ocho.*
          Eight including me. There's—there're seven brothers and me, there's eight of us.
Dr. Ortiz: *¿Y de chiquitos trabajaban ustedes?*
          And as children did you all work?

Complication 2

Norma: *Pues yo sí. Siempre yo creo que le ayudé a mi mamá. Siempre cuando yo ya pude, siempre yo le ayudaba a mi mamá pos que a una cosa y a otra. Y ellos se vinieron—hubo un tiempo que se vinieron para un lado de la costa, para Nayarit, que cortaban tabaco y todo eso. Yo me acuerdo, estaba chiquilla y yo les ayudaba. Ya después—ya después nos regresamos para allá y pues ya fui teniendo a mis hermanos y todo y pues yo le ayudaba nomás a mi mamá en la casa a batallar con los chiquillos, que a lavar pues allá puro lavar a mano. Uno le ayudaba a lavar y todo, y pues nomás en eso.*
          Well I did. I think I always helped my mom. Always, when I was able to, I would always help my mom doing one thing or another. And they came—there was a time when they came to one side of the coast, to Nayarit, that they would chop tobacco and all of that. I remember, I was little and I would help them. Then after—then after we returned from there and well I began

to have my brothers and everything and well I would just help my mom at home to deal with the little ones, wash well, over there it was all hand washing. One would help with washing and everything, and well just that.

Resolution

Norma: *Ya después cuando crecí, pues, yo me fui muy chiquilla con mi esposo. Yo me casé de—me fui con él cuando iba a ajustar doce años.*

Then after when I grew up, well, I left young with my husband. I got married at—I left with him when I was about to turn twelve.

Dr. Ortiz: *¿Doce? [Con tono de sorpresa].*

Twelve? [With a tone of surprise].

Norma: *Doce años y pues ya.*

Twelve years old and that's it.

Evaluation

Norma: *Se puede decir que ya toda mi adolescencia la pasé con viejo y hasta ahí pues ya. Porque mi hija la más grande la tuve cuando iba a ajustar 13 años.*

You can say that all my adolescence I was with the old man and that's that. Because my eldest daughter, I had her when I was about to turn thirteen years old.

At the opening, Norma only suggests that she realizes how much she despaired as a child on reflection. Since she does not offer any specific details, the doctor asks a few specific questions—whether her parents lived with her, and whether she worked during her childhood, which ultimately elicits more details. Getting up and getting her a tissue in between these questions shows a gesture of attentiveness and *simpatía*. The question about working demonstrates transcultural knowledge that a doctor ignorant of rural Mexico would not have. In fact, rural immigrants from socioeconomically disadvantaged families often worked as children. Norma stopped going to school by the second grade. While he demonstrates surprise that his patient married at the age of twelve—an extreme case among his patients—Dr. Ortiz approaches her leaving school to work with an equanimity that normalizes the history. Here he uses his socioeconomic and cultural awareness to establish effective transcultural communication.

Norma unfolds various details that are interrelated as part of her narrative, yet she both begins and ends by describing working from a young age to help her mother. The complications involve her father's absence, their financial struggles, and working during childhood. The resolution in the patient's story, marrying at age twelve, is not necessarily a "resolution" to her problems but rather a conclusion to or a result of that part of her story. In this case, the conclusion indicates the end of her childhood. Later in the interview, the doctor asks Norma about her marriage, and she reveals that her husband was twenty-two when they married and that he was controlling and abusive to her for many years. When they came to the US, their relationship improved, although they still had problems.

For most patients, the sociodevelopmental history elicits unfortunate stories, and many become emotional. Both patients featured in the last two examples shed tears as they told their stories. Such patient–doctor interaction is complex. Carlat (2012) explains that it is usually a mistake to try to comfort patients as one would a loved one. He recommends that health care professionals maintain their distance, offer a tissue, wait empathetically, and ask patients how they feel. These practitioner expectations in a professional setting are problematized when language and cultural barriers and socioeconomic status that have long marginalized patients are involved. Patients relay childhood struggles as well as social isolation, poor working conditions, discrimination, and dislocation upon immigration to the US. It is well documented that struggles like discrimination and marginalization directly affect the mental health of Latino/as in the US (López and Carrillo 2001). Latino/a patients are less likely to seek mental health care than, for instance, non-Hispanic whites, in part because it is challenging to find Spanish-speaking practitioners (López and Carrillo 2001). If Dr. Ortiz maintained a strict professional distance such as Carlat calls for, his patients might feel that he has assimilated to the norms of US doctors and aligns with the majority society and not the patients'. Instead, the doctor in this study achieves a balance between professional distance and familiarity, as evidenced through his language choice.

Dr. Ortiz adapts the interviews using his awareness of the circumstances of Latino/as in the Central Valley. He does not treat his patients as victims or as a friend would, but he demonstrates that he's their ally; for instance, he offers personal advice, as illustrated in chapter 3, on small talk. He shows empathy in reacting to patients' heartbreaking stories by displaying gestural (frowning, expressing sadness) and verbal affect, saying, for instance, "*qué difícil*" "how difficult," "*qué triste*" "how sad," and at times offering encouraging remarks. However, he also continues to ask questions to collect the information he needs. This consistency helps maintain the appropriate professional distance that a clinical relationship requires. Assuming this social role helps make the setting less threatening and more trustworthy, which ultimately encourages patients to tell their stories. Trust plays a particular role in screening for psychiatric disorders, which follows the section on sociodevelopmental history.

Screening for Psychiatric Disorders

Screening is a very medically oriented section of the interview. The patients answer in short responses (yes/no) to a quick survey designed to identify mood disorders (e.g., depression), appetite, energy levels, anxiety, obsessive disorders, and suicidal thoughts. The screening functions to collect relevant information that helps determine whether the patient should seek further psychiatric care.

As the doctor begins this part of the interview, he first lets the patients know about the structure of the questions (directions) and how they should respond (interpretation). He usually tells patients that there are about twenty questions, information he often has already provided but now repeats. The function of these instructions is to prepare patients for the mechanical feel of the numerous and quick questions. By warning patients of the structure of this section of the interview, Dr. Ortiz helps preserve the rapport he has built with them, and they are more likely to understand the necessity of such structured questions with preparation.

The screening of Alma, a female patient in her mid-sixties (#2), goes smoothly:

Instructions

Dr. Ortiz: *Le voy a hacer unas preguntas y me contesta sí o no.*
I am going to ask you some questions and you answer with yes or no.

Short Responses

Dr. Ortiz: *¿Durante las últimas dos semanas, ha estado deprimida la mayor parte del día casi todos los días?*
In the past two weeks, have you been depressed most of the day almost every day?

Alma: *Dos semanas. Casi. ¿Cómo le dijera? Entre sí y entre no. Como sí.*
Two weeks. Sort of. How could I say it? Between yes and no. Like yes.

Dr. Ortiz: *Mhm. A ratos sí, a ratos no.*
Mhm. At times yes, sometimes no.

Alma: *Sí.*
Yes.

Dr. Ortiz: *¿En las últimas dos semanas, le ha bajado el interés en las cosas que antes hacía?*
In the past two weeks, has your interest in things you would find interesting before decreased?

Alma: *Uhm, no, no. Antes, sí lo tenía.*

        Uhm, no, no. Before, I did have it [decreased interest].

Dr. Ortiz: *¿Sí?*

        Yes?

Alma: *Antes, pero ahorita ya no.*

        Before, but not now anymore.

Short Responses and Personal Exchanges

Dr. Ortiz: *¿Durante el mes pasado, ha hecho algunas cosas muchas veces seguidas sin controlarse? Por ejemplo, lavarse las manos y volvérselas a lavar y volvérselas a lavar.*

        During the past month, have you done some things repeatedly without control? For example, washing your hands once and then doing it again and again?

Alma: *[Silencio]*

Dr. Ortiz: *Varias veces seguidas.*

        Several consecutive times.

Alma: *Sí me las lavo seguido, sí. A la mejor la nuera también necesita asistencia psiquiátrica, de donde*

        Yes I do wash them often. Maybe my daughter-in-law needs psychiatric attention, from where.

Dr. Ortiz: *Pues sí, que le ayuden a controlarse.*

        Well, yes so they can help her control herself.

Alma: *Porque ella, este, pues*

        Because she, umm, well

While her answers are short, the patient adds personal exchanges to contextualize her responses and to engage in interpersonal interactions with the doctor (for instance, when she mentions her daughter-in-law), which is typical among the twenty-three patients. Most deviate from the "yes/no" responses to a certain extent by offering personal exchanges or (short) narratives, recounts, and anecdotes in addition to their short responses. As figure 2 illustrates, very few patients did not deviate to some extent. The doctor rarely initiates these deviations.

Deviations typically occur toward the middle and end of the screening; toward the beginning of this structural component, I mainly find short responses. Patients begin by answering the questions as instructed, but they switch to more socially oriented discourse once they seem more at ease. They react to the switch in the "field" (meaning the topic of conversation) from a more socially oriented field to a more medically oriented field through these deviations.

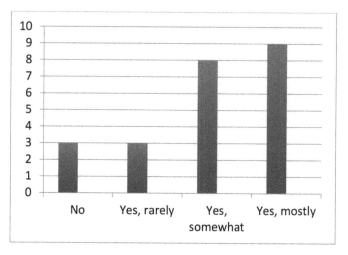

FIGURE 2. Deviations from short responses

The doctor does not remind patients who deviate from their short responses of the instructions he has given them initially. Had he done so, the patients would probably perceive this as rude, which could result in disruption of their rapport and of the comfort of the setting that had been created up until this point of the interview. Instead, he adjusts the interview according to the style in which patients answer the questions, such as acknowledging that Patient 2 may be correct about her daughter-in-law. This local accommodation to these specific patients is another indicator of the transcultural expertise of Dr. Ortiz.

Conclusions

This chapter has drawn from genre theory to describe the structural constituents of the psychiatric interview for a local community, as represented in the sample of Dr. Ortiz's interviews with his Spanish-speaking patients. The analysis suggests that the guidelines that textbooks offer for conducting interviews may not be specific enough for practitioners who serve culturally and linguistically diverse groups. Any live interview, because it involves real, dynamic speakers, is co-constructed and culturally and socially negotiated.

The chapter reveals recurrent subgenres within the schematic structures of the psychiatric interview. These include instructions, personal exchanges, and short responses, as well as specific subgenres for telling stories. Even more significantly, it describes the type of interpersonal trust that Dr. Ortiz aims to build with his patients, with personal exchanges particular evidence of this trust. Small talk and personal exchanges are important interactions in medical discourse, as research shows that they help doctors understand patients' lives and encourage patient participation (Cordella 2004).

In telling stories related to their sociodevelopmental history and the history of their present illness, patients use narratives with schematic patterns similar to those that Labov and Waletzky identify (1997). In the more elaborate stories, beyond the schematic structures, I was also able to look at how patients used phases in developing their stories. Other story genres that patients resorted to were recounts and anecdotes. Patients reconstruct their experiences through their stories, sometimes with the doctor's active support by means of specific questions that elicit more information, and sometimes with nods and other signals of listening. Dr. Ortiz uses his transcultural expertise to co-construct these stories, which are a key element during psychiatric interviews.

The structural components of the psychiatric interview as a macrogenre reveal the organization of the discourse from an ideational perspective. Ideational language allows us to look at the representation of experience; in this case, the doctor has certain goals he needs to meet with the patient's collaboration (Martin and White 2005). However, looking closer at patients' responses and the doctor's response reveals plenty of variation at a more interpersonal level, as both interlocutors deviate from short responses to personal exchanges. Therefore, the interview is composed of a macrogenre with specific structural components and subgenres found within these components. When considering the interviews from an ideational level, it is clear that the structural components have an overall organization based on the doctor's predetermined questions. However, in relation to the interpersonal level, pragmatic phases are distinct for each patient–doctor interaction, which vary according to many factors involved in the dialogue. The doctor continually makes local accommodations, which he can do because of his transcultural expertise. Chapter 4, which analyzes register, addresses this interpersonal level in greater detail, inspecting the tenor component and the interpersonal metafunction, for example, the relationship between the interlocutors.

In this chapter, I have sought to draw attention to what patients and the doctor do with the discourse, such that these data can influence the dialogue about transcultural communication in health care. The achievement of productive interviews like the ones Dr. Ortiz conducts reflects a complex interaction of subgenres in meaning-making. One of the primary goals of this chapter has been to consider the psychiatric interview as a configuration of meanings composed of specific schematic structures and, within these, different subgenres. The doctor controls the overall schematic components because of his power role. He determines the switch from one generic component to the next, and the patient expects him to do so. On the other hand, the patients, not the doctor, produce the subgenres and, in particular, the ones used for telling stories. In this way, Dr. Ortiz's rural Mexican patients create and negotiate meaning in the psychiatric interview to shed light on their (often underrepresented) discourse. This focus directly contrasts with the perspectives of common training materials about psychiatric interviews, which focus on what the doctors should and should not do and give little consideration to what patients do. Clearly, the creation and negotiation of patients in this context is a key element of completing the interview. More discourse-focused research that raises awareness of patient language use would be a step toward improving communication with patients. Since research has so little information about Spanish-language interviews, it is crucial to supplement psychiatry manuals and textbooks with actual contextualized interactions. To gain such data and have a more complete picture of psychiatric interviews that is inclusive of the voices of Spanish-speaking patients, further collaborations between linguists/discourse analysts and medical providers are needed.

Insights for Medical Practitioners and Interpreters

- In the history-oriented sections of the interviews (Present Illness and Sociodevelopmental), patients typically tell their stories using narrative or recount structures. An explicit awareness of how people tell their stories during various sections of the medical interviews is useful for developing interactional skills such as knowing when patients have completed their stories or when they may need more probing.
- Dr. Ortiz nourishes patients' narratives and is a co-constructor of these stories by actively or passively guiding the patient. In cases where he takes a more active role, he uses his transcultural knowledge to probe key details with sensitivity, for instance, when he asks patients whether they lived with both parents, whether they worked as children, whether they are caring (emotionally or financially) for an elderly parent, or whether they are separated from family members. Dr. Ortiz draws from his knowledge on the range of situations of rural Mexican patients to pose effective questions, which proves crucial to eliciting pertinent information. This is one of the reasons why hiring and recruiting providers who share ethnicity with their patients to medical programs is critical.

- Dr. Ortiz is flexible in collecting patient data during different parts of the interview and accommodates the interview when deviations occur. Patients deviate at times because they want to give more context to their answers, and the doctor not only approves of this changes but also deviates from his protocol. Even though in some cases patients offer data out of order, he adapts to the patient's structure, and yet he still collects the information he needs. This flexibility is an example of transcultural communication, which is particularly important when dealing with patients across classes. Given his awareness of the speaking practices of some Latino/as, he makes language choices that are respectful and thus helpful in a psychiatric assessment.

- The doctor achieves *simpatía* through numerous gestures throughout his interviews, including greeting the patient and walking with them to the exam room. This initial greeting is particularly crucial given that it is the doctor's first time meeting with these patients. Dr. Ortiz accepts patients' conversational offerings, even in the most structured part of the interview, and is attentive to patients' emotional needs, making courtesy gestures such as giving patients a tissue when they are visibly saddened. He achieves *simpatía* by acknowledging people's painful experiences at times through silence, through a break in the interview, or by displaying knowledge of the complex and challenging circumstances of rural immigrants from Mexico.

CHAPTER 3

Hacer Plática

Small Talk Subgenres

MAKING SMALL TALK during a medical interaction is crucial for creating a comfortable environment and establishing an interpersonal relationship, which promotes patient adherence to care. Through small talk, the interlocutors have the opportunity to get to know each other better.

Small talk is a conversation that the interlocutors mutually recognize as affirmative or prosocial but that may not serve any instrumental goal. It may occur during an action or as a prelude to a conversation that has a more instrumental goal.

Small talk offers an opportunity to bring the "life world" into the clinical visit (Mishler 1984). Further, it not only promotes the social connection between doctor and patient but also can readily become "big" talk as it covers information with medical ramifications (Ragan 2000). For instance, discussing social or familial topics can lead to environmental or medical information that can inform the doctor's recommendations and improve patient interactions (Coupland 2000). Ragan (2000) finds that patients whose doctors engage in small talk are more likely to cooperate with recommendations after the visit. For these reasons, Coupland (2000) and Ragan challenge the "smallness" of small talk. As Ragan says, "No talk in any context can be considered 'small'" because the relationships such conversations build are "inextricable features of every encounter" (282). Coupland suggests that "the solidarity and social support [small talk] achieves, in itself, can reasonably be thought of as part of [medical] 'treatment'" (22). Thus, in this work, the term *small talk* does not convey insignificance but is instead used to capture the type of social interactions that can take place in a professional context.

Small talk can include "joking, self-deprecation, laughter, complimenting, displaying modesty, and using reported speech" to indicate affinity and connection (Maynard and Hudak 2008, 673). Daniel Carlat explains in his widely used psychiatry textbook, *The Psychiatric Interview,* that he employs small talk to put patients "at ease." It is a way, he writes, of undermining the "projection" that psychiatrists are "mysterious, silent types who busily scrutinize patient's smallest gestures" (Carlat 2012, l2o). David Hayes-Bautista, an MD, professor at UCLA, and leading expert on Latino health care, puts greater emphasis on small talk, saying that discussion of nonmedical topics that are culturally relevant "help[s] me in many cases to break the ice and form a common bond" (Hayes-Bautista and Chiprut 2008, 9).

Small talk overlaps with central Latino values: *personalismo,* meaning value of a personal relationship, and *simpatía,* referring to friendliness and the avoiding of interpersonal conflict (Caballero 2011; Cordella 2004; G. Flores 2000). *Personalismo* refers to prioritizing an interpersonal relationship over an institutional one. In medical contexts, it requires showing genuine interest in the person beyond their medical condition, and requires small talk (Caballero 2011; G. Flores 2000). *Simpatía* can be supported by informal greetings, respectful language, allowing the patient to answer, avoiding jargon, and choosing colloquialisms (Cordella 2004). These values heavily intersect; one difference is that *simpatía* is a broader concept than *personalismo.* Because *personalismo* is more specific to small talk, this chapter focuses on how *personalismo* takes place in doctor–patient interactions.

The literature on small talk has mostly focused on English-language speakers (Coupland 2000; ten Have 1991; Maynard and Hudak 2008; Ragan 2000), but acceptable topics can vary by culture and language. Carlat recommends that psychiatrists engage in small talk about the weather and "difficulties arriving at the office" (2012, 20), although the latter may not be as relevant in cities that are easier to navigate or in areas with less traffic than the Boston metropolitan area, where he lives and works. Dr. Hayes-Bautista writes of using his "knowledge of and firsthand experiences with Mexican customs, national and religious holidays, and Mexico's political, educational, and health care systems" in small talk (Hayes-Bautista and Chiprut 2008, 9). A joke may be hard to translate since jokes are culturally informed, and small talk will be different between speakers of a dominant language in a particular culture than between speakers of a minority language.

Given that empirical evidence shows that interpersonal interactions can influence Latino/as' adherence to medical treatment and continuity of care, focusing on interpersonal interactions during medical interactions sheds light on a pressing challenge in Latino health care (Cordella 2004; Flynn et al. 2015). Latino/as are less likely to have continuity of care than non-Latino whites across various medical specialties (Zuvekas and Taliaferro 2003) and specifically after an initial visit to a psychologist (Alegría et al. 2008; Dingfelder 2005; Wassertheil-Smoller et al. 2014). Latino/as feel profiled and discriminated against in medical encounters (Barr and Wanat 2005; Martínez 2010, 2011). Feeling disrespected and mistreated and experiencing poor communication with providers affects follow-up care (Betancourt et al. 2011; Blanchard and Lurie 2004). A perceived lack of *personalismo* can negatively impact Latino/a patients' satisfaction and follow-up care (G. Flores 2000).

On the flipside, when doctors emphasize friendliness, they can better influence patients' decisions and foster patient compliance and patient satisfaction with their encounter (Cordella 2004). Cordella (2004) highlights the need to train more doctors to use what she calls a "fellow human" voice, meaning showing empathy to encourage patients to tell their stories. Similarly, Flynn and collaborators (2015) propose that improving health practitioners' interpersonal skills can improve continuity of care while reducing health disparities affecting Latino/as.

Even though small talk plays a crucial role in health care delivery, few studies have focused on how these everyday interactions unfold in authentic medical encounters. The few that have shed light on these interpersonal interactions have been mostly on English-language interactions. This chapter offers a systematic analysis of small talk in Spanish between a doctor and his patients by using genre, as in chapter 2, to examine how their interactions unfold. Genre analysis, within the systemic functional linguistics (SFL) approach, is useful here for discussing the macrolanguage in small talk, including cultural expectations and practice (Magaña 2018a). Dr. Ortiz has transcultural competency: the ability to communicate in linguistically and culturally appropriate ways with his Spanish-speaking patients. This competency is critical to his effective employment of small talk. Thus, by analyzing how these interactions unfold at the level of genre, this chapter points to specific examples of *personalismo* and explores how meaning is constructed through transcultural interactions.

Determining the boundaries of small talk, which is more socially oriented, and medical talk, which is more goal-oriented, is not always clear-cut (ten Have 1991). In psychiatric interviews, interactions about patients' personal experiences may seem socially oriented but simultaneously inform the doctor's medical goals. In this book, I consider small talk to be any type of social interaction that helps foster an interpersonal relationship between Dr. Ortiz and his patient. These interactions are usually not part of the doctor's explicit agenda since they deviate from the forms that guide the interview, but they may inform his diagnosis. Because these are the doctor's first psychiatric interviews with each patient, building an interpersonal relationship, many times through small talk, is essential.

Small Talk Genres

On average there were 3.5 small talk exchanges per interview. Systematic inspection of the transcripts of the twenty-three interviews reveals that small talk has the most significant presence toward the beginning of the interview, though it can occur at any time. The doctor often uses information from the demographic questions (which appear toward the beginning of the interview) to make an interpersonal comment. When patients initiate these social conversations, they more often occur at the beginning of the interview as well.

The linguistic devices for making small talk include, from most to least common, brief personal exchanges, recounts, and gossip. Each serves the function of building trust and solidarity in distinct ways, as the next sections discuss.

Personal Exchanges

Personal exchanges are spontaneous moments of social interaction that derive naturally from the task-oriented topics. They include compliments, humor, personal advice, and cultural topics in common between patients and doctor (traveling to Mexico, Mexican food and traditions, the experiences of Mexicans in the US, etc.), and self-disclosure by the doctor.

Cultural Topics

When collecting demographic information from patients, the doctor usually demonstrates interest in patients' hometowns in Mexico and initiates personal exchanges. In example (1), when Ricardo (a male in his late forties, #21) says he was born in the state of Oaxaca, the doctor asks for more specific details about where precisely he was born. This leads to a discussion of its proximity to "the city," and a self-disclosure by the doctor:

1) Cultural topics

Dr. Ortiz:	*¿En dónde nació [patient's name]?*
	Where were you born [patient's name]?
Ricardo:	*Uhm, yo soy del estado de Oaxaca.*
	Uhm, I'm from the state of Oaxaca.
Dr. Ortiz:	*¿Qué parte de Oaxaca?*
	What part of Oaxaca?
Ricardo:	*Uhm, en [name of town].*
	Uhm, in [name of town].
Dr. Ortiz:	*¿Eso está cerca de la costa?*
	Is that close to the coast?
Ricardo:	*No, está cerca de la ciudad.*
	No, it's close to the city.
Dr. Ortiz:	*¿Cerca de la ciudad?*
	Close to the city?
Ricardo:	*Sí.*
	Yes.
Dr. Ortiz:	*Mi ciudad favorita de México.*
	[That's] my favorite city in Mexico.
Ricardo:	*¿Oh sí?*
	Really?
Dr. Ortiz:	*A mí me encanta ir a Oaxaca. Yo soy del D. F.*
	I love going to Oaxaca. I'm from Mexico City.
Ricardo:	*Del D. F., cerquita de ahí.*
	From Mexico City, close by.
Dr. Ortiz:	*Sí, ahorita ya está a cuatro horas.*
	Yes, right now it's four hours away.
Ricardo:	*Cuatro o cinco horas.*
	Four or five hours [away].

At first neither the doctor nor Ricardo explicitly mentions the name of the city near the patient's hometown they are referring to. They call it "the city" and share an understanding of which city it is (Oaxaca).

The doctor continues to gather demographic information but then refers again to the shared cultural knowledge of the city familiar to both of them:

2) Cultural topics

Short Responses and Personal Exchanges

Dr. Ortiz: *¿Cuándo nació?*
            When were you born?
Ricardo: *Uhm, soy del* [birth date].
            Uhm, I was born on [birth date].
Dr. Ortiz: *A comer tlayudas al mercado.*
            Let's eat *tlayudas* at the market [some time].
Ricardo: Yeah, *y los estos* . . .
            Yeah, and the, those . . .
Dr. Ortiz: *Chapulines.*
            Grasshoppers.
Ricardo: *Chapulines, tasajos.*
            Grasshoppers, jerked beef.
Dr. Ortiz: *Ya me dio hambre. ¿En qué trabaja?*
            Now I'm hungry. What's your job?

This example demonstrates how the doctor demonstrates *personalismo* while accomplishing his medical goals. He parallels the interview questions with spontaneous comments and questions about Oaxaca and its food, and even jokingly says that talking about food has made him hungry. The personal exchange is not disruptive to the information the doctor is gathering (Maynard and Hudak 2008). While the statement "let's eat" and the reference to "those" grasshoppers as if they were right there might sound odd in English, as if the two grown men were engaging in preschool-style imagination games, in the context of the interaction, it merely suggests warmth and engagement. The interlocutors in this context are two immigrant Mexican men, one of whom may not have the means to visit Mexico. They use the immediacy of the Spanish language through the present tense as a way to bond over the immigrant experience. These exchanges encourage the patient to be at ease, and his facial expressions and body language evidence this.

Chapulines (grasshoppers) are a signature Oaxacan dish. There is a fair amount of significance to referencing a dish that many non-Mexicans consider strange. Through his use of a shared cultural affinity, the doctor signals his identification with the patient and strives to build solidarity. Their interaction is an example of transcultural communication, not only because the doctor knows about the patient's local traditions but also because he decides to use this knowledge strategically during the interview to identify with the patient.

Another form of knowledge the doctor uses is positive statements about the Mexican immigrant community. For example, when he asks patients about drug use and they say no, he mentions, in some cases, that drug use is low among Mexican immigrant communities. He comments on their strong work ethic and good parenting (specifically the dedication of Mexican mothers to their children). In the following example, he comments on how hard it is to work in the fields, where the local Mexican immigrant community is overrepresented, in his interview with Pilar (a woman in her thirties, #5):

3) Cultural topics
Dr. Ortiz: *¿Y en qué trabaja su marido?*
            What does your husband do for work?
Pilar: *Está en el campo.*
            He works in the fields.
Dr. Ortiz: *Mhm. Pesadísimo, ¿no?*
            It's hefty work, no?
Pilar: *¿Mande?*
            Excuse me?
Dr. Ortiz: *Es pesado.*
            It's heavy work.
Pilar: *Pues, sí. Sí es pesado.*
            Well, yes. It is heavy work.

In this personal exchange, the doctor is aiming to show his *personalismo* and to help make the patient feel more relaxed and less threatened by the medical environment. Pilar is not as talkative as other patients. This example is a shorter small talk interaction than most.

Humor draws on culture in a very specific way. It is culturally embedded, and to effectively participate in a humorous exchange, one needs to be aware of the culture's social norms or risk offending another person.

Humor

Humor is a discursive device that aids in making small talk (Maynard and Hudak 2008) and that can be used to minimize potential face threat, which refers to an act that challenges an interlocutor's self-image (Brown and Levinson 1987). Eggins and Slade propose that humor "enable[s] interactants to speak 'off the record,' to make light of what is perhaps quite serious to them, in other words, to say things without strict accountability, either to themselves or to others" (2005, 156). In the medical context, humor mitigates patients' psychological stress and decreases their anxiety (Ragan 2000). In his conversation with Ricardo about *chapulines,* the doctor used a joke, "now I'm hungry," to transition back to the demographic questions and away from discussing the market in his favorite city.

The doctor frequently uses humor when asking about serious topics such as religion, marital status, and substance abuse to create a more relaxed environment. For instance, the doctor jokingly comments on patients' answers about religious affiliation, as in this example with Cesar (a man in his thirties, #22):

4) Humor

Short Response

Dr. Ortiz: *¿Religión?*
Religion?

Cesar: *Católico.*
Catholic.

Personal Exchange

Dr. Ortiz: *¿De a de veras?*
For real?

Cesar: *Uhm, parte.* [smiling]
Uhm, partly.

The patient's smile suggests that he is very engaged with Dr. Ortiz at this point. This may stem from the doctor's informality and lack of piety in saying "for real?" regarding religious affiliation; it may stem from a feeling that the doctor has correctly identified that Cesar does not necessarily follow all the tenets of the Catholic Church.

The doctor asked three out of the twenty-three patients about the veracity of their religious affiliation, and in each case, the patient seemed amused and intrigued by the question. Transcultural understanding has to exist between both speakers for the humor to work in these interactions. Both speakers know that among Mexicans, following Catholic traditions and attending church regularly are culturally well-regarded practices. At the same time, not following the Church's edicts is socially sanctioned. Given this transcultural understanding, the doctor uses his authoritative figure to bring out the guilt in the "partly" Catholic patient in a friendly and lighthearted way.

Patients also initiate humor. In the following interaction with Trinidad (a woman in her sixties, #11), the patient's choice of words, by including "just," invites a humorous interaction:

5) Humor

Dr. Ortiz:	*¿Casada? ¿Cuántas veces se ha casado?*
	Married? How many times have you been married?
Trinidad:	*Mhm, nada más una.*
	Mhm, just once.
Dr. Ortiz:	*¿Nada más una?*
	Just once?
Trinidad:	*Nada más una. ¿Se imagina usted que me vuelva a casar? ¡Con la muerte; eso es lo que va a pasar!*
	Just once. Could you imagine if I remarried? [I'll remarry] with death; that's what will happen!
Dr. Ortiz:	*Qué dramática.*
	So dramatic.
Trinidad:	[Laughs]
Dr. Ortiz:	[Giggles]

The use of "just" by the patient invites the humorous interaction, whereas "once" alone would not. The doctor's question, "just once?" implies that he recognizes she is indicating she would not have any problem finding a second husband if she wanted one, and it leads her to reveal her traditional marriage values (i.e., one marriage for life). This is a serious topic that the patient can discuss with more ease through humor. The doctor's gentle ribbing when he says she is dramatic to reference marrying death reveals his (opposing) views on marriage/remarriage. It is this opposing view that creates the humor in this interaction. As Eggins and Slade explain, humor can depend on difference, as it occurs in contexts that involve "conflict, tension, and contradiction" (2005, 167).

Humor eases the threat of the unfamiliar environment by making a conversational deviation from the interview through personal exchanges. The doctor and patients in this study use humor to connect at an interpersonal level and mediate their power differences (Ragan 2000). He used humor with both men and women. By contrast, compliments also generate laughter, but he gives them only to women.

Compliments

The doctor compliments his female patients on their devotion to their children, perseverance, healthy lifestyles, and youthful appearance. He does this in a respectful manner and during the appropriate contexts, which shows *personalismo,* such as with Amalia (seventies, #20):

6) Compliments

Dr. Ortiz: *¿En 1937 nació?*
            You were born in 1937?
Amalia: *Sí. Estoy muy viejita.*
            Yes. I'm very old.
Dr. Ortiz: *Se ve como de cincuenta, como de mi edad.*
            You look like a fifty-year-old, like my age.
Amalia: *Tengo setenta y dos años. [Risas] Bien acabados.*
            I'm seventy-two years old. [Giggles] So worn out.

In the course of this exchange, the doctor makes a self-disclosure of his own age. As well, while the patient laughs, the doctor does not. Both of these indicate his *personalismo* in that he means his compliments seriously, and he is willing to talk about his own age.

Personal Advice

The doctor offers advice that does not pertain to potential psychiatric disorders. For instance, he tells patients that it is good to pursue a higher education, how to obtain prescription eyeglasses, and how to seek US citizenship. In a number of these cases, he discusses his own experiences concerning this advice. For example, in this exchange with María (a woman in her mid-forties, #18), he encourages her to use English even if it is not perfect:

7) Personal Advice
Short Response
Dr. Ortiz: *¿Qué tal habla el inglés?*
            How well do you speak English?
María: *Uhm, lo entiendo a unos, pero pa' hablarlo me da vergüenza.*
            Uhm, I understand it with some, but I get embarrassed speaking it.
Personal Exchanges
Dr. Ortiz: *¿Pero por qué?*
            But why?
María: *Sí, me pongo a veces con unas personas a practicarlo, pero no.*
            Tengo que . . . yo sé que tengo que ponerme las pilas.
            I do practice it with some people, but not [enough]. I have to . . .
            I know I have to get on it.
Dr. Ortiz: *¿Va a la escuela o fue?*
            Do you go or did you go to school?

María: *Uhm, fui; fui dos años en Los Ángeles.*

             Uhm, I went, I went for two years in Los Angeles.

Dr. Ortiz: *Mhm. ¿Llegó a Los Ángeles primero?*

             Mhm. You came to Los Angeles first?

María: *Uhm, en [city name] viví.*

             Uhm, I lived in [city name].

Dr. Ortiz: *En [city name]. No, háblelo, háblelo, no pasa nada. Así como los gringos hablan feo cuando hablan el español . . .*

             In [city name]. Speak it, speak it, it's okay. Just like the gringos, they speak badly when they speak Spanish.

María: *Yo sé.*

             I know.

Dr. Ortiz: *Nosotros podemos hablar feo cuando hablamos el inglés.*

             We can also speak English even if it's badly spoken.

María: *Yo sé.*

             I know.

Dr. Ortiz: *Y no pasa nada. Pero lo entienden.*

             And it's okay. Because they understand.

María: *Sí.*

             Yes.

By using the first-person plural, *nosotros,* the doctor includes himself. As he implies, like María, he learned English as a second language during his adulthood. The personal advice here shows a strong sense of cultural and interpersonal solidarity and reflects bicultural mentoring. Self-disclosure also suggests solidarity.

Self-Disclosure by the Doctor and Other Topics of Small Talk

The doctor often self-discloses as a way to make small talk and to show *personalismo.* As described in example 6, he references his own age in talking about his patients, or, as in example 1, he refers to where he grew up in talking about his patients' hometown. Another time his patient mentions that she works at a gym, and the doctor asks which one. When she tells him, the doctor tells her that he used to be a member.

In a medical interview, participants usually have a nonreciprocal-asymmetrical relationship. In this case, the doctor knows plenty about the patients from their records and, through the interview, is collecting even more information, whereas the patients know little about him. Thus, self-disclosure by the doctor makes the interview more socially symmetrical. The doctor also uses self-disclosure to offer indirect advice to patients. For instance, after one of the patients tells the doctor about shoulder and arm pain, the doctor tells him about his own shoulder surgery and suggests that he communicate his complaints to his general practitioner.

Other small talk topics arise incidentally. For example, when his desk shakes during one interview because it is not very stable, the doctor mentions an earthquake in Los Angeles as a way to inform the patient of recent news. Patients often mention the educational successes of their children as a way to make small talk, and the doctor shows keen interest.

Recounts

Recounts function to share experiences, but unlike narratives, they have no resolutions. In this genre, interlocutors discuss a sequence of events without significant disruption (Martin and Rose 2008). The schematic structure is as follows:

(orientation) ^ record of events ^ (reorientation)

In the following case, the doctor initiates small talk by asking Miguel (a man in his mid-forties, #7), who has symptoms of depression, about visiting Mexico. This topic of conversation is common to both doctor and patient, as both are from Mexico. When the doctor asks how the patient is able to visit Mexico, the patient tells his story using a recount. I have divided it into its structural components below.

8) Recount

Orientation

Dr. Ortiz: *¿Todavía vas [a México]?*
 Do you still go [to Mexico]?

Miguel: *Yo voy.*
 I go.

Dr. Ortiz: *Órale, ¿cómo le haces? Yo no he podido ir.*
 Right on, how do you do it? I haven't been able to go.

Miguel: *Pues así. Pido prestado por ahí porque no me ajusta el dinero.*
 Well like this. I borrow to go if I don't have enough money.

Record of Events

Miguel: *Sí, es que tengo a mis padres allá y a mi madre le pegó el embolio, entonces por eso es que me hice para allá, pues [para] mirarlos.*

> *Pues, a ver si yo quiero ir este año y le digo a mi señora, se me*
> *hace que se me va a hacer de agua. No tengo dinero, pero espere-*
> *mos en Dios en que esto va tarde y ya, pues, juntar una feriecita*
> *para ir a visitarlos.*
> Yeah, it's just that my parents are there and my mother had an
> embolism, then that's why I want to go, well to see them. Well
> let's, if I want to go this year and I tell my lady, I think it's not
> going to go through. I don't have money, but God willing that
> this happens late and that's that, well, gather some bucks to go
> visit them.

Reorientation

Miguel: *Pero pues a veces me dan ganas y a veces no, por problemas.*
But well, sometimes I feel like going and sometimes I don't,
because of problems.

Miguel reveals that he borrows money from others to visit his ailing parents
in Mexico; this is the orientation of his story. The record of events (or problems) includes his sick parents, the geographic distance between him and his
parents, and the financial hardships that affect his travel. In the reorientation stage, the speaker returns to the present moment, where he evaluates his
choices and explains the difficulty of his situation, acknowledging that sometimes he doesn't go even when he wants to. The complications go unresolved
in the story, which they would not in a narrative.

The doctor's statement "*órale*" "right on" is colloquial, and it elicits small
talk, as does his self-disclosure about his own difficulties traveling to Mexico.
Miguel then reciprocates the self-disclosure, revealing critical information
about his finances and family health that may relate to his psychiatric health.
This is an example of how the doctor's *personalismo* enhances his understanding of his patients.

As this example demonstrates, small talk facilitates the medical goals of
the encounter (Coupland 2000; Ragan 2000; Stivers and Heritage 2001). As
the patient in example 8 reveals his financial situation and the stress caused by
his ailing parents, the doctor gains insight into the patient's potential underly-
ing triggers of depression.

Gossip

Small talk can also take the form of gossip. Gossip involves sharing judgments
about others' culturally significant behavior to create a connection between

interlocutors (Eggins and Slade 2005). Eggins and Slade (2005) propose that gossip conforms to the following generic structure:

third-person focus ^ substantiating behavior ^ pejorative evaluation

These stages may be recursive. Optional components include probing for more details and wrapping up by summarizing the theme or behavior (Eggins and Slade 2005).

In one case, the doctor and Alma (a woman in her mid-sixties, #2) engage in gossip about the patient's daughter-in-law during the screening section of the interview. The patient has revealed problems she has with the daughter-in-law, who lives in the same household, throughout the interview. According to the patient, her daughter-in-law's substantiating behavior, meaning the evidence that prompts the gossip, includes having friends who encourage her to go out, going out for as many as three hours at a time, expecting the patient to watch her kids, talking back to the patient (e.g., after the patient tells her not to go out), and going out shopping soon after having a C-section. The patient's gender-role values clash with those of her daughter-in-law. In this case, the patient believes that mothers should be more focused on their children and thus should spend more time at home. By providing the doctor this information about her daughter-in-law, the patient is trying to get to know the doctor better and therefore to establish solidarity with him, to establish that they share the same views of motherhood (Eggins and Slade 2005, 285).

Much of the time, the doctor does not respond directly to the gossip. He maintains eye contact and uses continuer markers such as "aha" and "hmm." However, in the next example, the doctor becomes a more active participant in the gossip. This interaction follows the portion of Alma's interview described in chapter 2, in which she says that she washes her hands compulsively, and then says that her daughter-in-law does as well. Then she brings up her daughter-in-law again:

9) Gossip

Third-Person Focus

Alma: *A la mejor la nuera también necesita asistencia psiquiátrica, de donde . . .*
         Maybe my daughter-in-law needs psychiatric attention, from where . . .

Dr. Ortiz: *Pues, sí, pa' que le ayuden a controlarse.*
         Well, yes, so they can help her control herself.

Alma: *Porque ella, este, pues . . .*
         Because she, umm, well . . .

Evaluation

Dr. Ortiz: *A ponerse en su lugar.*
Set her straight.

Alma: *Sí.*
Yes.

Dr. Ortiz: *O necesita que la eduquen.*
Or she needs to be taught to behave.

Alma: *Uyy, mi hijo le tiene miedo.*
Yikes, my son is scared of her.

Probing

Dr. Ortiz: *¿Sí?*
Really?

Evaluation

Alma: *El le tiene miedo a ella. Hasta para que me hable a veces.*
He is scared of her. Even when he wants to talk to me.

Wrap-up

Dr. Ortiz: *Así pasa.*
That's how it goes.

The doctor's reference to how medical professionals could "help her control herself" is a professional observation. His evaluation "*A ponerse en su lugar*" "Set her straight" has an ambiguous meaning. It is unclear whether the doctor refers here to addressing a psychiatric disorder that the daughter-in-law might have or to addressing her disrespectful behavior toward Alma. Thus, the doctor aligns himself with Alma in an effort to bond with her: "*necesita que la eduquen*" "she needs to be taught to show more respect" (to her mother-in-law / the patient). Like her condemnation of her daughter-in-law's outings, her reference to her son being "scared" of his wife may suggest a traditional understanding of gender roles, as it seems to indicate that a man can be excused for intimidating his wife—but never the other way around. The doctor wraps up the gossip, saying "*Así pasa*" "That's how it goes," indicating that he recognizes those situations, but he does not offer any further judgment. This moves the conversation on from gossip and back to the interview questions.

In the following conversation, the doctor asks Ramón (mid-thirties, #13) about his marital status. This leads the patient to gossip briefly about his ex-wife:

10) Gossip

Dr. Ortiz: *¿Eres casado?*
Are you married?

Ramón: *No.*

Dr. Ortiz: *¿Has sido casado?*

            Have you been married?

Ramón: *En un tiempo, pero nomás un año duré.*

            Once I was, it only lasted a year.

Third-Person Focus and Substantiating Behavior

Ramón: *A la señora le gustaba andar con muchos hombres.*

            That woman liked being with many other men.

Evaluation

Dr. Ortiz: *Mientras sean dos o tres está bien, pero muchos no, ¿verdad?*

            As long as it's two or three it's fine, but not many, right?

Probing

Ramón: [Laughs] *Ta duro pa' encontrar mujeres horita, ¿edá?*

            It's hard to find [good] women these days, right?

Evaluation

Dr. Ortiz: *'Ta duro.*

            It's hard.

Probing

Ramón: *No sabes en qué te vas a meter.*

            You don't know what you're getting yourself into [when you get involved with women].

Wrap-Up

Dr. Ortiz: *Ándale.*

            Exactly.

The patient uses his masculinity to seek a bond with the doctor. The doctor, by agreeing in part with Ramón, shows *personalismo* in choosing to close their interpersonal distance.

During the interviews, Dr. Ortiz never initiates gossip, but he generally responds at least somewhat positively when his patients initiate it. He also is always the one to wrap up the gossip and move on in the interview. The doctor's willingness to gossip involves stepping outside what may be considered expected behavior from him as a medical provider. Thus, he prioritizes bonding with his patients over professional norms. Dr. Ortiz might be compromising his own point of view in order to bond with patients. Another critical point is that the patients give the doctor this opportunity or invitation to engage with them in gossip. Therefore, this example shows us both an insight into the types of discourse choices that a doctor can make to achieve transcultural communication and the ways in which patients invite providers to bond.

Conclusions

This chapter offered a linguistic description of small talk during psychiatric interactions between a doctor and his patients using genre analysis. Small talk is dynamic and spontaneous and can occur throughout the interviews in distinct discursive forms. Small talk interactions are essential in medical consultations, as they help doctors understand the context of their patients' lives and encourage patients to participate actively in the medical interview (Cordella 2004). Engaging in small talk with patients and learning about their "lifeworld" is a way to not only learn about patients but also to improve their health care and education (Stivers and Heritage 2001). In a psychiatric interview, small talk is vital for setting a comfortable environment for the patient, an essential step given that the interaction involves sensitive topics. Small talk interactions are departures from the traditional restrictions of the interview genre. Still, the doctor uses them to build rapport and establish an interpersonal and a transcultural relationship with patients. He employs transculturally appropriate strategies showing his *personalismo*; most of the strategies are socially oriented and interpersonal, but they play a crucial role in completing the medically oriented task.

The transcultural elements that play a critical role in communicating with these patients include the doctor's knowledge about the patient's cultural norms. Dr. Ortiz deploys this knowledge, for instance, when he uses humor, self-discloses, offers personal advice, and compliments patients, all of which are culturally informed language choices and rooted in the construct of *personalismo*. Based on individual interactions, he decides when it is appropriate to engage in small talk and about what topic and how to demonstrate transcultural competency. At times, he goes against his own social norms to establish a professional bond with the patient, as we saw when the doctor broke with the gendered expectation that Mexican men should not gossip.

Genre analysis reveals that small talk is not a simplified social exchange but rather a complex interpersonal activity that can take the form of different genres: recounts, gossip, and personal exchanges. This analysis offered an explicit description of these interactions and illustrated how transcultural communication and interpersonal communication intersect with each other. This chapter has aimed to promote sociolinguistic awareness of the explicit forms and the transcultural content of small talk to illustrate examples of patient-centered consultations and how *personalismo* unfolds across numerous interactions. Chapter 4 further explores the social and power roles of each interlocutor during the psychiatric interviews by analyzing the register of these interactions with a particular focus on the relationship between the participants.

Insights for Medical Practitioners and Interpreters

- Small talk has an important place in medical interviews because it contributes to patient adherence and continuity of care. It is particularly crucial for Latino/a patients, who are less likely than non-Hispanic white patients to feel safe during their health care consultations. Small talk is an integral element in medical communication that helps mediate the power, professional, and experience inequalities of the participants (Cordella 2000). By revealing personal information about himself, offering patients advice, and demonstrating interest in patients' social lives, the doctor in this study presents himself as a fellow human being and thus empowers patients.

- Small talk during the beginning of the interview helps create a more familiar atmosphere. Small talk topics include the doctor's comments on Mexican cities, foods, or customs. His humor, compliments, personal advice, self-disclosure, agreeing (at least in part) with gossip, and expressing positive views of the contribution of Latino/as in the US all serve the same purpose. Advice that is not medically related also has a positive impact.

- Through the doctor's small talk, we witness a local adaptation of a professional genre in service of a particular community, which serves as an explicit example of how to achieve transcultural competence and precisely how to convey *personalismo*. It is crucial for practitioners to learn to use these authentic interactions to supplement the guidance offered in psychiatric textbooks, since these textbooks may not capture diverse and local communities, such as rural Spanish speakers in the US. For instance, in medical Spanish courses, we should offer models of transcultural competency based on actual interactions and highlight the language choices that promote effective communication with patients. Genre analysis is particularly suitable as a pedagogical tool because it can help learners become more explicitly aware of how communication is negotiated and how specific language choices are culturally informed.

CHAPTER 4

Register of the Psychiatric Interview

Interlocutors, Power, and Solidarity

THIS CHAPTER FOCUSES on register analysis of the psychiatric interviews as a means to explore their context. I draw, here, on Halliday's (1978) approach to register within systemic functional linguistics (SFL). Halliday described field, tenor, and mode as the main variables in a particular context that influence language choices. Register refers to the situational factors related to the context of communication and is composed of three variables: field (which refers to topic), tenor (which relates to interlocutors), and mode (which refers to the role of the language). Most of this chapter focuses on tenor rather than on field or mode because it is the language variable that enables me to explore the relationship between doctor and patients carefully.

Studies that have inspected doctor–patient questions and their intersection with power dynamics have examined English-language interactions in places where English is the dominant language (Ainsworth-Vaughn 1998; Frankel 1990; West 1984). The research I present examines interactions in Spanish that took place in the US. Not only is Spanish a minority language in this context, but the specific variety that patients speak is also stigmatized. Given this strong contrast between the populations being studied, it would be interesting to explore the differences and similarities in the patterns found in the literature.

This chapter considers the interview discourse in even greater detail than previous chapters because, according to the levels of language stratification in

SFL, register is more discursively "concrete" than genre. Whereas genre allows us to reveal the context of culture in a text, register reveals the context of the situation. The difference between the two is that register explains how specific variables function, whereas genre offers a broader way to look at medical language. One of the register variables, tenor, allows me to closely inspect the social roles of the interlocutors and to consider how these affect the language choices in a bilingual setting. This chapter also describes in detail the variables that make up tenor, affect, contact, and power. Through register analysis, I explore the power variable concerning the interlocutors, using descriptive statistics characterizing the questions that each party poses and who controls the conversation based on each party's word count. The goals of this chapter are to describe some of the idiosyncrasies that characterize this register and to reveal how the power relationship between the interlocutors is evidenced through language.

The Field of the Psychiatric Interview

Field refers to the subject matter of the text (e.g., climate change) or the topic of conversation in spoken language (e.g., weather, sports). The field of psychiatric interviews is mental health history. Analysis of field captures precisely how these topics get constructed through language. For instance, analysis of field raises awareness of the level of formality that participants employ. When interlocutors share technical expertise, the field may be very formal. However, medical experts rightly advise doctors to avoid speaking to patients in the same way they would speak to other doctors. Even when a doctor and patient speak the same language, jargon can impede communication (Carlat 2012). Unfortunately, doctors use jargon with patients, particularly when they want to name specific symptoms and syndromes, to index that they identify as part of a rarified expert group, and to index their elite status and exclude others; patients misunderstand their doctors as a result (Wodak 1996). Using a technical register can compromise the health of patients, since patients may not seek clarification, especially if they fear that asking for clarification will anger the doctor and compromise treatment (Wodak 1996).

Neither Dr. Ortiz nor his patients generally use a technical register in the consultations this study analyzes. As illustrated in the results of genre analysis, most of the questions the doctor poses use everyday language. Patients tend to describe their medical conditions using everyday language and rarely employ specific medical terms. For example, Martín, a male patient in his early fifties (#17), describes his symptoms thus:

1) Everyday language

Martín: *Me estoy despertando y cuando me despierto pues bien sobresal-*
            tado, bien—o sea bien nervioso, bien angustiado porque sé que
            tengo que hacer muchas cosas y no las estoy haciendo. O sea, sí
            me doy cuenta de que tengo que hacer las cosas y no las hago.

            I am waking up [at night], and when I fully wake up, well, I get
            very startled, very like, very nervous, really worried, because I
            know that I have many things to do, and I am not doing them. I
            mean, I do realize that I have things to do, but I don't do them.

The doctor similarly avoids technical terms. He also checks with a patient
if he does use a technical term, as, for example, when he says to Pilar, a female
patient in her mid-thirties (#5): "*¿Ha tenido ataques de pánico? ¿Sabe lo que*
es un ataque te pánico?" "Have you had panic attacks? Do you know what a
panic attack is?" The patient shakes her head, and the doctor explains, listing
three symptoms:

2) Everyday language

Dr. Ortiz: *Que siente que se le sale el corazón y empieza a sudar como si le*
            fuera a dar un ataque y siente que se va a morir.

            You feel that your heart is going to burst and you start sweat-
            ing as if you were going to get a heart attack, and you feel that
            you're going to die.

The patient finds this explanation illuminating, and she responds: "*Una vez me*
pasó algo, pero no sé si sería eso." "Something happened to me once, but I'm
not sure what it was." She describes her experience; the doctor listens and then
confirms that indeed it may have been a panic attack.

While the doctor shows his sensitivity to the issue of clarity concerning Pilar, clarification requests are the most common type of questions that
patients ask. For example, Roberto, a male patient in his early forties (#8),
seeks clarification by asking "*¿Perdón?*" when the doctor asks him whether
he perspires. The doctor changes the form of the word from "*¿Sudoración?*"
to "*¿Suda?*" In switching from the noun, he switches from asking Roberto to
supply an item for a list of symptoms to asking, with less formality, "Do you
sweat?" Roberto understands and answers affirmatively.

In other cases, Dr. Ortiz replaces technical language with colloquialisms.
As he told me in our interview, he does this not to make the medical term
more accessible but to be culturally appropriate. For instance, he uses more
culturally relevant terms when the technical terms are taboo. For example

in asking Érica, a female patient in her mid-thirties (#19), about the method of delivery of her child, he substitutes a colloquial term for "vaginal birth" (*parto vaginal*), "*nacer por abajo*," which means literally "to be born from down there." He makes no such substitution for cesarean ("*cesárea*"). In this case, the patient would understand "*parto vaginal*," but it may have made her slightly uncomfortable to be asked a question that has an explicit reference to her sexual organs. The colloquial phrase functions as a euphemism and as a way to maintain *respeto*. This example illustrates Dr. Ortiz's transcultural competence in recognizing the potential problem and knowing an alternative linguistic choice.

Dr. Ortiz tries to pose questions that are comprehensible and accessible for all patients who have been exposed to different registers of Spanish than he. For instance, patients are less familiar with more technical registers of Spanish than the doctor is. While such a gap exists between doctors and almost all patients, Dr. Ortiz's patients have a wider gap due to sociocultural factors, especially their drastic differences in education levels. The doctor is strategic in avoiding technical terminology not only for comprehension reasons but also for cultural reasons.

The Mode of the Psychiatric Interview

Mode refers to the level of aural and visual contact or distance between interlocutors and the level of formality. The former generally determines feedback response time. For example, we would expect immediate feedback between interlocutors who are friends having an informal, face-to-face conversation. At the other extreme, a book offers no visual or aural contact between interlocutors—that is, the writer and reader—which delays feedback significantly. These two extremes are also proposed as the extremes of formality. We find formal language in a book and informal language in face-to-face friendly interaction.

The mode of the psychiatric interview belongs somewhere along the formal and informal language continuum, but the interaction is face-to-face. The psychiatric interview also has a specific generic structure that the doctor follows using a prepared questionnaire, as discussed in chapter 2. This structure makes the interaction more synoptic given its organization and its less dynamic nature than, for example, a conversation between friends. The exchange is somewhat predictable, whereas informal language is more spontaneous. However, Dr. Ortiz's language suggests that he strives to create a relaxed atmosphere. Through the use of nonstandard grammar, nonstandard pronunciations, spontaneity, and colloquialisms, he aims to make the context more comfortable for the patient. The small talk I described in chapter 3 is one of Dr. Ortiz's strategies for realizing this familiarity. In analyzing mode, I look more closely at these strategies, which the doctor employs subtly to negotiate the formal nature of the interview.

Using colloquialisms makes the message accessible to the patient while creating a more symmetrical interaction and is a way to aim to create *confianza* (Cordella 2000, 43). Using familiar language also increases reports of socially undesirable behaviors (Carlat 2012). Daniel Carlat (2012), a psychiatry expert, advises practitioners to use "shooting up" instead of the more clinical "intravenous drug use." However, doctors who train in the US and conduct Spanish-language interviews rarely receive comparable information for interactions in Spanish (Ortega et al. 2020). This lack of knowledge can have communicative consequences given that *confianza* is an essential cultural construct among Latino/as. Unlike the colloquialisms in "field," where the function was to avoid technical terms for comprehension reasons or taboo terms to prevent embarrassment, mode encompasses how colloquialisms add informality to the language. The doctor employs these lexical items to display solidarity with his patients and to have a stronger connection with them; in other words, to create *confianza*. Table 3 offers a sample list of colloquialisms that the doctor uses during the consultations and their standard counterparts.

The doctor uses both the colloquialisms and the more formal terms. For example, when collecting the demographic data, he usually uses *trabaja* (work), but a few instances later in the interviews he uses the colloquial *chamba* (grind) to create more informality. Everyday terms for drinking alcohol, such as *chupe* (drinking), *chelas* (beer), or *cheves* (beer), appear only in interviews with men. Mexican men tend to use these slang words in informal conversations with other men, and the doctor introduces them to add informality to the interaction and to create *confianza*.

Patients sometimes use colloquialisms that the doctor does not understand. For example, Érica, a female patient in her mid-thirties (#19), reveals that she has dealt with depression and describes changes in her eating habits (eating more junk food than before her depression). She uses a regionalism, *guzguera* (junk food), which the doctor did not understand. She clarifies by offering some specific examples—"*galletas, sabritas*" "cookies, chips"—and a synonym—"*chucherías*" "junk food." The doctor is interested in the terminology, and he asks about it:

TABLE 3. Colloquialisms and standard synonyms

COLLOQUIALISM	STANDARD SYNONYM	STANDARD FORM TRANSLATION
a lo bestia	salvajemente/ exageradamente	savagely
ahorita	en este momento	right now
ándale	de acuerdo	right
chamba	trabajo	job
chance	oportunidad	chance
chela	cerveza	beer
cheves	cervezas	beers
chilango	de la ciudad de México	from Mexico City
chupe	tomar alcohol	to drink alcohol
cuidarse	usar protección	to use protection
dar	golpear	to hit
entrarle duro	excederse de	to overindulge
hacerle a la jugada	jugarse	to gamble
jalar	funcionar	to function
machín	macho	macho
meterse drogas	usar drogas	to use drugs
ponerse loco	emocionarse	to get excited
ponerse bien jarra	emborracharse	to get drunk
soda	refresco	soda
tristón	triste	sad

3) Colloquialism

Dr. Ortiz:	*¿Así les dicen en Zacatecas?*
	Is what you call them in Zacatecas?
Érica:	*¿Eh?*
	Huh?
Dr. Ortiz:	*¿O aquí?*
	Or here?
Érica:	*Pues, yo no sé la verdad.*
	Well, the truth is I don't really know.

Zacatecas is the patient's birthplace. The doctor's interest in dialectal uses of Spanish is evidence that he has sociolinguistic and dialectal awareness. He does not treat any dialect as superior to another but instead implies that they are all distinct ways of making meaning. At the same time, he demonstrates interest in further developing his transcultural competence, adding new colloquial terms to his register while empowering the patient by treating her as the expert in Spanish spoken in Zacatecas.

The doctor's interest in developing awareness of the colloquialisms people use is crucial because it may reveal how populations understand particular conditions or symptoms (Cabassa et al. 2008; Lackey 2008). For example, a reference to depression includes colloquialisms such as "feeling blue," but this does not work in Spanish. On the other hand, Spanish has specific colloquial references that are not used in English, as discussed below.

In line with acknowledging the use of colloquialisms to create a patient-centered approach, Lackey (2008) examines how thirty-eight Mexican immigrant men identify depression and perceived causes and remedies. When asked about colloquial terminology for depression, common responses include *agüitado* (depressive attitude), *achicopalado* (depressed with an emphasis on lack of energy), *estar cabizbajo* (being sad and lacking energy), *andar sacado de onda* (distracted by thoughts/confused and troubled), and *estar desganado* (lacking interest and energy to do anything).

When describing their depression and anxiety symptoms, patients in this study use the following descriptions,[1] summarized and translated in table 4.

These descriptions of depression and anxiety symptoms include colloquialisms and folkloric explanations of illnesses (meaning popular knowledge passed through generations) that are similar to those reported in the literature on Latino mental health, such as *nervios* and *susto* (fright) (De la Torre and Estrada 2015; Y. Flores 2013). Yvette Flores provides an explanatory model that uses a cultural perspective in Latino health care, stating that Latino/as believe that diseases are caused by an "imbalance from or within relationships, or imbalance between the heart, mind, and body" (2013, 53). Thus, some Latino/as may ascribe depression to *nervios,* a broad category of mental health issues attributed to interpersonal imbalance (Y. Flores 2013; Guarnaccia et al. 1989). *Nerves* is a close translation, but it does not encompass the whole. Flores describes the causes of *nervios* as "related to an individual not being true to his or her word, not living with integrity," as well as having conflict in important relationships; the symptoms, "bouts of crying, tension, listlessness, loss of appetite, irritability and sadness," would generally meet contemporary Western medical understandings of depression (54).

---

1. These descriptions may have multiple meanings and translations, but the translation provided here refers to the meaning most closely associated with the context in which it was used.

TABLE 4. Patients' descriptions of depression and anxiety symptoms

PATIENTS' DESCRIPTION	TRANSLATION
me agarran los nervios	I get *nervios* (nerves)
me da susto	I get *susto* (fright)
me apuro	I worry
me dio pánico	I panicked
me da desesperación	I get frenzied
me empiezo a sentir caliente	I start to feel hot
me entra angustia/ angustiado/a	I get anguished
me entra depresión	I get depressed
me entra nervios	I get *nervios* (nerves)
mi estómago me brinca mucho	my stomach "jumps" a lot
mi estómago me tiembla	my stomach trembles
me falta el aire	I am short of breath
me siento alterada	I feel anxious
me siento angustiado/a	I feel anguish
me siento decaído/a	I feel weak
me siento desesperada/ me desespero	I feel frenzied
me siento desguanzada (no tener fuerza)	I feel weak
me siento entumida/o	I feel numb
me siento mareada/o	I feel dizzy
me siento nervioso/a	I feel nervous
me siento sobresaltado/a	I feel startled
me pega mucha taquicardia	I get a lot of tachycardia
se me acelera el corazón	my heart starts rushing
siento aguados mis pies	my feet feel weak
tengo miedo	I feel scared

Adopting local colloquialisms can empower patients to speak about their issues during their medical encounters despite stigma (Carlat 2012). De la Torre explains that "understanding the cultural nuances and idiosyncratic belief structures of [a] group is critical to interpreting [its] language" (De la Torre and Estrada 2015, 131).

Misunderstandings can occur if a medical provider is unaware of the culturally based interpretation of illnesses and symptoms (De la Torre and Estrada 2015). Dr. Ortiz is familiar with these cultural interpretations and uses this knowledge to gather more information from patients or to explain a symptom or disease that a patient does not understand. For example, Ricardo is a patient in his late forties (#21). He had described dealing with symptoms of depression. The doctor asks him, "*¿Además de que de repente se deprime y anda triste y eso, le da como ansiedad?*" ("Besides suddenly getting depressed and sad, do you get like anxiety?"). The patient does not understand *ansiedad* (anxiety). Dr. Ortiz clarifies, with alternative descriptions of the term using *angustia* (anguish) and *nervios,* which is sufficient for Ricardo to say that he has experienced it. As with several other patients, the doctor does not assume that Ricardo knows what a panic attack is, and he asks. Since the patient says no, Dr. Ortiz explains: "*Que la gente de repente empieza a sudar y siente que se va a desmayar y le late muy fuerte el corazón*" ("When people suddenly start to sweat and feel that they are going to faint, and their heart starts to beat very fast"). Ricardo is able to answer this question in the affirmative.

Similarly, patients may not use the terminology the doctor proposes but instead contribute their own description. In the example below, when the doctor asks the patient, Cesar (mid-thirties, #22), whether he has felt depressed (*deprimido*), Cesar does not use this term and instead offers his own, *decaído* (downhearted):

4) Colloquialism

Dr. Ortiz: *¿Has estado constantemente deprimido la mayor parte del tiempo durante las últimas 2 semanas?*
Have you continuously been depressed most of the time during the last two weeks?

Cesar: *Yo diría que sí, como **decaído** sí.*
I would say, yes, like downhearted, yes.

Patients' registers point to an understanding of diseases and symptoms that require in-depth knowledge of Spanish. Beyond his use of formal or technical of Spanish registers, Dr. Ortiz is successful in diagnosing his patients because he is familiar with colloquial or folkloric knowledge. It may be possible for doctors with genuine interest to learn about these culturally specific conceptualizations of health and synonyms for medical terms to offer patient-centered care, however.

The Tenor of the Psychiatric Interview

Tenor refers to the relationship between interlocutors and its levels of formality (e.g., student and instructor, mother and daughter, close friends).

Informal Language   **Formal Language**

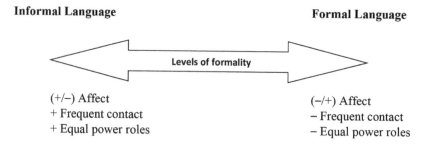

(+/−) Affect   (−/+) Affect
+ Frequent contact   − Frequent contact
+ Equal power roles   − Equal power roles

FIGURE 3. Formality language levels of affect, frequency of contact, and power

Adapted from María Cecilia Colombi, 2003, "Un Enfoque Funcional para la Enseñanza del Lenguaje Expositivo," in *Mi Lengua: Spanish as a Heritage Language in the United States, Research and Practice,* edited by Ana Roca and Cecilia Colombi, 78–95 (Washington, DC: Georgetown University Press).

Doctors and patients obviously have a more formal relationship than most family members or close friends. One of the first linguists to offer a detailed analysis of tenor, Cate Poynton (1989) proposed that it consists of three variables that influence the formality or informality of the language: power, contact, and affect. For instance, in an interaction where the interlocutors' power is equal and where the various elements of contact generate intimacy and positive affect, such as an interaction between two friends, they typically use language characterized by informality. At the other extreme, power and a lack of positive affect can overwhelm even frequent contact, as in exchanges between a police officer and a civilian. Figure 3 illustrates the role of power, affect, and frequency of contact according to a continuum of (in)formality levels.

The variables of register work interdependently and, at times, in overlapping ways. In building a network of options for tenor, Poynton proposes that these options are all "culturally meaningful alternatives" that produce "culturally significant communicative behavior" (1989, 79). In analyzing the tenor of the psychiatric interviews using the dimensions of contact, power, and affective involvement, we find a complex positioning for each interlocutor and variable.

Contact

Contact contrasts intimacy with social distance. Frequency of interaction, the amount of time speakers have known each other, the number of capacities by which interlocutors relate to each other, and whether the interaction is task-oriented or people-oriented all affect contact (Poynton 1989).

The patients in this study are being screened for psychiatric disorders, and if any disorder is suspected, they are to be referred to a specialist for further screening and, if needed, longer-term care. They have no particular expectation of additional encounters with Dr. Ortiz, and they have never met him before. Their time together is limited. Thus, neither interlocutor has an incentive to invest much in building a relationship or much time to begin to create one. There is no role diversification—the doctor and patients do not know each other in other capacities. The orientation is complex. It is mainly task-oriented, yet the task—screening patients—imposes a human orientation on the interview. The doctor tries to connect with the patients as a fellow human who shares their minority status as Latino/as and who understands the immigration necessity of Mexicans. Thus, he incorporates colloquialisms and makes small talk, all while demonstrating transcultural competency.

Affect

Affect can be either positive or negative, and unlike contact or power, it may be absent. Contact and power also influence affect. When some combination of intimacy, frequency of interaction, long periods together, role diversification, human orientation, and equal power produces an informal situation, speakers are more likely to express their attitudes than when speaking in more formal situations.

The concept of "affect" has been further developed into an SFL-based approach, the appraisal framework. This approach characterizes affect as the attitude of the interlocutors, its change throughout an exchange, and the tone of dialogic interactions. Attitude includes emotional reactions to one another's ideas, and judgment, positive or negative, of the other conversant's behavior.

Using the appraisal system, I found that the doctor generally shows positive judgment of the patients' statements, which serves to bring him closer to patients. For example, when patients say that their family or friends are supportive, or how proud they are of their children, the doctor says something like "está bien" "that's good," "muy bien" "very good," or "¡qué bueno!" "how great!" When a male patient in his early forties praises a doctor he had seen, who was known to Dr. Ortiz, he says, "¡qué bueno!" The patient agrees, saying, "Sí, es muy bueno" "Yes, he is really good." By contrast, patients do not display judgment about the information the doctor provides or the questions he asks, although they do display judgment of others in their lives who are not present.

The doctor rarely displays emotion, but patients do, as they are speaking about their feelings. For example, Érica (#19) expresses a good deal of emotion when describing her experience of being told that her baby had severe congenital disabilities when she was pregnant. She references insecurity, uneasiness, shock, and unhappiness:

6) Affect

Érica: *Cuando me estaban diciendo, yo ya* **no quise saber nada,** *no quise saber ni qué iba a hacer, ni que, nada, les dije, "saben qué yo no quiero saber nada."* **Me quedé en shock.** *O sea,* **me sentí muy mal.** When they were saying this to me, I didn't want to know anything else. I didn't want to know what I was going to do, nothing at all. I told them, "you know what, I don't want to know anything." I was in shock. I mean, I felt horrible.

She references happiness, as well:

Érica: *. . . porque ya* **estaba ilusionada,** *ya le empezaba a comprar ropita. Lo sentía que se movía, le cantaba, pos, estaba* **bien ilusionada.** *Incluso mi niño, tengo un niño de cinco años, y el niño pos* **estaba bien contento,** *y ya cuando me dijeron eso pos yo* **me sentí bien mal** *porque primero no quería y después ya que estaba* **ilusionada.**

. . . because I was excited. I had already bought clothes for the baby. I felt him moving, I sang to him. I was really excited. Even my kid, I have a five-year-old boy, and the kid was really happy, and then when they told me that, well, I felt very horrible, because at first I didn't want to be pregnant but later I was thrilled.

In this case, we find a contrast concerning the patient's feelings. On one hand, Érica says she was pleased about the pregnancy. She intensifies it with adverbs (*bien* and *muy*) and through repetition. On the other hand, she expresses distress after the complications with her unborn child and the loss of this child by using negative affect and again intensifying these feelings.

Analysis of affect reveals a great deal about the power relationship between doctor and patient. Specifically, it indicates which interlocutor has the right or obligation to reveal his or her feelings (the patient in this case) and which one is more likely to display judgment about the interlocutor's statements (the doctor).

Power

Power is a variable of tenor and ranges from unequal to equal with the following factors contributing to this equality: authority, status, and expertise. It functions strongly during patient interviews. Patients in this study are Mexican rural immigrants or Mexican Americans with rural heritage. While the doctor is also Mexican, unlike the patients he was socialized in an urban middle-class area of Mexico and received a high level of education. The doctor gains power because of his socioeconomic status, cultural background, and expertise. He controls the structure of the interview as a token of his medical knowledge.

To further inspect the power variable between doctor and patients, this chapter considers what occurs in the discourse that offers insights as to these social positionings. In a medical interaction, ways of claiming power include interruptions, posing questions, and holding the floor (Ainsworth-Vaughn 1998). Interruptions are a sign of power because they challenge a speaker's right to finish his or her thought while having the floor. On the other hand, speakers who pose a question claim the right to choose the next speaker and the topic (Ainsworth-Vaughn 1998). The following sections offer descriptive statistics assessments of which interlocutor asks more questions, how much time each speaker holds the floor, and who interrupts whom and how.

Power and Questions

The following clinical definition of an assessment interview appears in an influential textbook on conducting psychiatric interviews:

> An interview represents a verbal and nonverbal dialogue between two participants, whose behaviors affect each other's style of communication, resulting in specific patterns of interaction. In the interview one participant, who labels himself or herself as the "interviewer," attempts to achieve specific goals, while the other participant generally assumes the role of "answering the questions." (Shea 1998, 7)

In asking questions, one interlocutor takes the role of seeking information while the other gives information requested. The patient is a passive interlocutor; the health practitioner is the active one. These roles add to the doctor's power as an expert and restrict the patient. Research has found that many patients feel intimidated or unable to ask questions during interviews (Frankel

1990; Katz et al. 2007). Being a clinic patient, having a temporary relationship with medical practitioners, and being financially disempowered instead of a private-practice patient who would have longer-term relationships with a practitioner and perhaps more financial resources affect speakers' power roles. In addition to these dimensions, being a member of a minority group contributes to asking few questions, probably a signal of the power of social distance (Ainsworth-Vaughn 1998; Eggly et al. 2011; Katz et al. 2007). Nonwhites and people with lower health literacy also tend to ask fewer questions than whites and those with higher levels of health literacy (Eggly et al. 2011; Katz et al. 2007; Menendez et al. 2017). Asking fewer questions contributes to health disparities in access to information because asking questions yields more information. Majority groups have other privileges that enhance their communication in medical institutions; for example, whites are more likely to be on a first-name basis with their doctors, a sign of informality (Ainsworth-Vaughn 1998). Patients in this study are being seen at a community clinic and not a private practice, and most have low health literacy levels, but they share ethnicity and language with the doctor.

A statistical description of the questions that Dr. Ortiz and his patients ask provides a concrete idea of the significance of questions in the psychiatric interview. It also provides a basis for comparing Dr. Ortiz's interviews with other research findings on patient–doctor interactions in other medical genres and distinct sociopolitical, linguistic, and cultural contexts. Before presenting the descriptive statistics on the questions asked, I explain the criteria I used to decide what to categorize as a question.

Question Criteria

I look at the entire discourse and context to determine what to consider a question. This perspective allows me to include indirect questions, statements that elicit an answer, and rhetorical questions that elicit responses. I include requests for clarification or information but exclude discourse markers such as *¿sí?* (yes?), *¿verdad?* (right?), and sometimes *¿no?* (no?) unless they elicit answers or are used to seek clarification. The count of questions does not include questions embedded in patients' narratives that are not directed to the physician. If an interlocutor said the same question twice with the second time functioning for emphasis, I counted it as one question rather than two. My sample contains words whose change in intonation was sufficient to form a question: for example, the doctor asking with a rising intonation, "*¿casada?*" (married?). These elided questions occur typically after the doctor has asked complete questions.

The data include requests for clarification even when these are formed as indirect questions because these utterances indicate that the patient is taking an active role in ensuring that she comprehends. For example, when one of the patients poses the indirect question "*No sé qué es ataques de pánico*" "I don't know what a panic attack is," the doctor answers the implicit question by describing a panic attack.

Some questions were rhetorical and functioned at times similar to a command; I included these as well when their function was to seek information, whether or not the other interlocutor provided it.

Descriptive Statistics for Questions

My criteria identified 1,576 total questions across twenty-one[2] patient interviews. On average, patients asked 3.9 percent of these, and the doctor 96.1 percent. The doctor averaged 84 questions per consultation; patients averaged 3.3 questions. The doctor's dominance parallels most of the previous findings on this topic. West (1984), who studied twenty-one encounters between white doctors and ten white patients and eleven African American patients in a family practice, found that patients asked 9 percent of the 838 total questions during their consultations. Cordella (2004) found that among twenty-two patients speaking to four doctors in an outpatient clinic in Chile in the dominant language, Spanish, patients asked 9.6 percent of the 394 total questions. Frankel (1990) found, in studying ten encounters in ambulatory care visits between patients and their long-term practitioners, that patients asked less than 1 percent of questions (total number of questions was not available). However, Frankel used a restrictive criterion for questions, which may tend to exclude more patient questions than doctor questions. Ainsworth-Vaughn's (1998) study examining forty encounters of patients and providers who were white and had a long-term relationship with their (white) physicians found that patients asked 39 percent of the 773 total questions. These findings are summarized in table 5.

The contrast between my results and other similar studies suggests that the type of medical setting in which the questioning occurs, the kind of relationship patients have with practitioners, and patients' socioeconomic status and

---

2. In this calculation I excluded two patients who had brought a family member to their consultation. Having a third party present completely changes the dynamic of an interaction, as seen in studies on interpreters (Davidson 2000, 2001; Angelelli 2004). Interestingly, patients in this study asked the most questions, at twenty-one and thirteen questions, not including their family members' questions. The sample, however, is too small to determine whether these findings are meaningful.

ethnicity all influence the number of questions patients will ask. The spectrum of results may suggest that patients in this study asked few questions in part because of their minority status in the US, their low socioeconomic and health literacy levels, and the clinical context of their visit. Ainsworth-Vaughn notes that "patients in subsidized clinics usually lack . . . shared interactional history and the fundamental reciprocity of full fees for medical services" that supports asking questions (1998, 97).

The types of questions patients pose were mainly clarification requests constructed through discourse markers (¿eh?), phrases (¿mandé? excuse me?) or indirect questions such as "Perdón, no entiendo" (Sorry, I don't understand). Even asking these, patients are deferential in and apologetic for making such requests, as shown in their openings: perdón (sorry), disculpe (forgive me; polite form), mande (excuse me but literally meaning "you're in charge"). Such questions usually led the doctor to clarify by rewording the question or giving examples.

I do not believe that the fact that patients ask only 3.3 questions on average suggests that Dr. Ortiz fails to create a trustworthy environment. He used small talk, colloquialisms, and showing respect, overall demonstrating transcultural competency. It may be that his patients would have asked fewer questions had he not used these techniques. The purpose of the interview, a preliminary psychiatric assessment, also likely discouraged queries, as patients would have the opportunity to ask questions of a long-term provider after the referral that the visit would facilitate. As Shea writes in her textbook, the goal of the psychiatric interview is "to gain a thorough and valid database in a limited amount of time while sensitively engaging with the patient"; answering questions is not the doctor's intent (1998, 7). Therefore, the specific genre of the interviews and its format may be another reason why there are fewer questions in the data.

Further, the number of questions asked in the interview is not the only indicator of the functioning of power in the interviews. Dr. Ortiz finds other ways to empower patients, as my analysis of holding the floor, interruptions, and discourse features to index solidarity shows.

Holding the Floor, Interruptions, and Power

Patients ask very few questions, and they do not switch topics or determine the next topic of conversation. Still, they hold the floor for most of the time during the psychiatric interviews. Who does the talking in a situation reveals information about the relationship between interlocutors, or tenor (Eggins

TABLE 5. Patient questions in studies on medical consultations and sample size

STUDY	PATIENTS' QUESTIONS (%)	TOTAL NUMBER OF QUESTIONS
Present study (2021)	3.9	1,576
West (1984)	9	838
Cordella (2004)	9.6	394
Frankel (1990)	1	not available
Ainsworth-Vaughn (1998)	38.7	773

2004). Cordella's (2004) study of patients in Chile found that patients held the floor about equally with doctors: doctors spoke about 583.1 words per consultation; patients spoke 587.4 words. She also notes that patients use an "initiator" voice to ask questions and to seek information about their health, and therefore that this voice provides patients one way of holding the floor and claiming their right to be heard. In Dr. Ortiz's interviews, patients do most of the talking, speaking 70.5 percent of the words, or an average of 2,550 words per consultation, while the doctor speaks 1,066 words per session (see table 6).

The range varied significantly: the least talkative patient spoke 1,079 words (the doctor spoke 963 words in that consultation), and the most talkative patient used almost six times that amount, at 6,250 words (the doctor spoke 1,152 words). Some patients were more concise in speaking than others, and some were initially reluctant to talk at all. Others wanted to share more of their stories during the discussion of their social development / childhood history and their clinical histories and to have a social conversation with the doctor.

Medical training aims to teach future doctors "to limit the flow of information without seeming insensitive and impatient" when patients are overly talkative (Carlat 2012, 39). Practitioners are advised to gently interrupt such patients. Interruptions are powerful discourse moves in the sense that they assert the exclusive right to speak. While interruptions may have little weight in informal interactions among friends, in a formal context where the speakers have little contact and unequal power relations, interruptions have more force. Research has documented that interruptions signal the power dynamics of the interlocutors in the patient–doctor relationship (Ainsworth-Vaughn 1998). Language interpreters recognize power dynamics in that they interrupt patients more often than they interrupt physicians (Davidson 1997).

Research also finds that interruptions can be dangerous in health care. In analyzing the discourse of emergency department patients, Slade and collaborators (2008) found that interruptions by clinicians led to fragmented stories, missing information, and delayed diagnosis. Clinicians who did not interrupt

TABLE 6. Words spoken by doctor and patients

PERSON	AVERAGE PER CONSULTATION	PERCENTAGE OF WORDS SPOKEN
Doctor	1,066	29.5
Patients	2,550	70.5
Total	**3,616**	**N/A**

their patients generated a feeling of ease in them that was conducive to good patient care. Erzinger's (1991) examination of a medical interview between a Hispanic patient and a doctor who spoke Spanish as a second language shows that because the doctor did not interrupt the patient, the interview had fewer awkward or clumsy interactional features than interactions in which doctors had interrupted more often.

When patients tell their stories, they are recreating their realities and accepting their illness (Ainsworth-Vaughn 1998). This means that the act of telling their stories is an integral part of their healing process. For these reasons, Ainsworth-Vaughn recommends that doctors not interrupt patients during their narration: "physicians can recognize important stories, cooperate with the telling, and learn a great deal about patient's specific needs in the process" (1998, 186).

As table 7 summarizes, the doctor interrupts patients six times on average per interview, a low number given the number of questions he is supposed to ask. He frequently interrupts to ask a follow-up question, to comment on a patient's response, or to offer clarification. Patients very rarely interrupt him, but when they do, it is usually to ask for clarification.

My interview with Dr. Ortiz revealed that his few interruptions are a deliberate strategy. He usually waits until patients finish speaking. Analysis of the interviews shows that he does not even interrupt when the patient deviates from the target question. For example, when patients offer details about their medical history as he collects demographic information, Dr. Ortiz deviates from the generic structure to accommodate them instead of interrupting and adhering to the prescribed order. He finishes collecting demographic information later in the interview. Minimizing interruptions in a medical consultation is a clear sign of showing *respeto* from both patients' and doctor's sides.

Dr. Ortiz did interrupt Trinidad, a female patient in her mid-sixties (#11):

7) Interruption

Dr. Ortiz: *¿Usted cuándo nació Trinidad?*
             When were you (formal) born, Trinidad?

TABLE 7. Interruptions by doctor and patients

PERSON	RAW NUMBER	AVERAGE PER INTERVIEW
Doctor	137	6
Patients	30	1.3

Trinidad: *Uuh, yo nací [fecha] del 44. Así es de que ya 65 años oiga.*
Oh wow, I was born on [date], 1944. So, yes, I'm already 65 years old, sir.

Dr. Ortiz: *Ándele.*
There you go.

Trinidad: *Ya me pesan los años, ya, ya, ya, ya no crea; ya le digo a mi hija—*
The years are taking a toll on me. I tell my daughter—

Dr. Ortiz: [interrupts] *¿Usted ya no trabaja tampoco?*
You don't work anymore either?

While the doctor maintains focus on the demographic questions instead of asking why Trinidad feels the years are taking a toll on her, he nonetheless transitions smoothly from her topic, her old age, to the likelihood that she no longer works because of her age. He also uses negative polarity, a polite form, to soften the question (asking with *respeto*).

Out of all patients, Alma, a patient in her mid-sixties (#2), is the most talkative. Dr. Ortiz interrupts her only three times:

8) Interruption

Alma: *Después me mandaron a esta clínica. Gracias a Dios aquí, este, la primera doctora que me atendió, luego, Lidia y Candy; sí iba a un programa ahí del diabetes. Y ahorita, este, gané las 17 libras, más como tres o cuatro libras más, ¿verdad?*
Afterward, they sent me to this clinic. Thank God for this, here, well, the first doctor that saw me, then Lidia and Candy; I was going to a diabetes program. And right now, I gained seventeen pounds, like three or four more pounds, right?

Dr. Ortiz: *¿Y en cuánto anda su azúcar?*
How is your sugar level?

The interruption follows several minutes in which the patient holds the floor. Dr. Ortiz's question is an effective transition from Alma's narrative because the question is related to the diabetes program she has just referenced. While the doctor interrupts, he nonetheless indicates that he is listening to the details of her story and is interested in them, and that therefore she is being heard. He uses the information the patients provide to pose a question when interrupting them and poses his question in a gentle way.

Conclusions

Register analysis has offered this study tools for systematically studying the linguistic options in a psychiatric interview more closely. This chapter has explored the factors that influence the language choices, the social context of the interaction, and the role of the interlocutors in terms of power, affective involvement, and solidarity. The power dynamic between doctors and patients is complex. Analysis of this sample of psychiatric interviews shows the workings of power and how they influence speakers' linguistic tools. The nonreciprocity of the roles of doctor and patient indicates the unequal power relations between the doctor and patients.

Nevertheless, Dr. Ortiz aims to empower his patients by minimizing interruptions and showing *respeto*. Even though he asks most of the questions, and therefore determines the topic of conversation, when the patients hold the floor the doctor only sporadically interrupts. When he does interrupt, he uses transitions and polite versions of questions to make the interruption smoother, which contrasts with the findings of other research on medical interactions (Davidson 1997; Slade et al. 2008; Wodak 1996).

Another idiosyncrasy that characterizes the register in the interviews is how the interlocutors use informal language. Typically in analyzing the tenor of doctors and patients using the dimensions of power, affect, and contact, we would expect to find formal language reflecting inequality in power. Doctors generally have power over their patients due to their expertise, socioeconomic status, education, and the relatively less powerful role of patients in this context. However, the interviews analyzed here show something different. Analysis of the everyday language used in the interviews reveals that the doctor replaces technical terms with familiar words to increase patients' comprehension. Although each interview has a structure, the doctor uses the more interpersonal sections of the interview to his advantage to add informality and to empower the patient. By using informal registers of speaking, such as colloquialisms, Dr. Ortiz aligns with patients, displays solidarity, and creates *confianza*.

On the other hand, patients' descriptions of depression and anxiety symptoms point to the importance of training practitioners to have colloquial and folkloric knowledge of health conceptualizations.

Insights for Medical Practitioners and Interpreters

- Having colloquial knowledge is essential for practitioners to offer patient-centered care. In mental health it is critical for providers also to have linguistic awareness of alternative and local-specific ways to ask about depression symptoms. There are cases where patients do not understand a medical term in Spanish that the doctor uses (e.g., *ansiedad* in example 1). Dr. Ortiz is still able to obtain relevant information from patients because he is equipped with alternative explanations for the medical terms, which at times entails culturally based or folkloric knowledge. Beyond language, the doctor's transcultural competency allows him to collect necessary information from patients. Given the value of having informal/colloquial knowledge for use in professional contexts, language classrooms on medical Spanish should teach the local varieties of the language (Ortega and Prada 2020), and doctors without cultural knowledge should be allotted extra time with their patients to obtain such knowledge.
- Colloquialisms can have multiple purposes. Not only can they aid in comprehending patients' health conceptualizations; they can also help create *confianza*. The doctor used his colloquial knowledge to bring up personal information such as his drinking habits casually. *Confianza* is not only a pivotal cultural construct for Latino/as but also an essential element of successful psychiatric interviews for any patient.
- The patients in this study asked very few questions. Research suggests that asking questions correlates with privilege (e.g., white middle-class patients ask numerous questions during interactions with their practitioners). It is crucial to continue working toward explicit strategies to encourage Latino/a patients, especially those of low socioeconomic status, to ask questions. These strategies can include (1) deliberately reminding them that they can and should ask questions and making it clear that this is not disrespectful, (2) giving them sample questions to ask, (3) periodically pausing to give them time to ask, and (4) asking them whether they have any questions during various moments of the interview. These are key ways to address health care disparities.

CHAPTER 5

Translanguaging in Health Care Interactions

IN ADDITION TO EMPLOYING STRATEGIES like small talk and colloquialisms, Dr. Ortiz mitigates the power between himself and his patients through translanguaging, which draws on both his bilingualism and his sociolinguistic awareness to accommodate patients and create *confianza*. Translanguaging is "not simply to a shift or shuttle between two languages, but [rather] the speakers' construction and use of original and complex interrelated discursive practices that cannot be easily assigned to one or another traditional definition of a language, but that makes up the speakers' complete language repertoire" (García and Wei 2014, 24). A translanguaging lens rejects the outsiders' perspective of languages as rigorously separate systems. Thus, adopting a translanguaging lens allows researchers to consider speakers' linguistic repertoire holistically because it considers languaging to be a unified collection of linguistic features in the speakers' languages "without regard for watchful adherence to the socially and politically defined boundaries of named (and usually national and state) languages" (Otheguy et al. 2015, 283).

A major feature of translanguaging is code-switching, which occurs when bilinguals alternate their languages, such as in the sentence "*Vivo con unos* [I live with some] roommates." During the interviews patients and the doctor code-switch for place and location names (Rite-Aid, Davis), eponyms (where brand names are often used generically, such as Kleenex and Pampers), and other foods and drinks (Sobe juices, Red Bulls, ice tea). It is a language practice in which bilinguals shift between the two languages effortlessly and naturally. Dr. Ortiz's effective medical Spanish reflects knowledge of which words his patients are likely to understand or even prefer in English.

Other bilingualism practices that translanguaging encompasses include the use of loanwords and semantic extension. These are a natural result of languages in contact, such as that between English and Spanish in the US. Because of the bilingual context in which Dr. Ortiz's interviews take place, English-language influence is common.

Loanwords are phonologically integrated into Spanish, and Spanish speakers in the US use many borrowed from English routinely. Indeed, Dr. Ortiz and his patients alike used loanwords such as *troca* (truck), *refil* (refill), *checar* (checkup), and *hobi* (hobby) in the interviews. Loanwords from English are considered colloquial and often carry stigma. In Spanish-language classrooms, students are typically told that they are incorrect, which stigmatizes communities of US Spanish speakers where these terms are common, ignores the realities of language use and its communicative function, and does not invite students to critically examine the role of prestige and appropriateness in language. Because of this, Spanish-language students often do not develop sociolinguistic awareness unless they take courses with specific sociolinguistics content (Martínez 2003), a significant point for instructors teaching medical Spanish.

Semantic extension, which also commonly occurs in bilingual contexts, refers to a word whose meaning may have been extended or changed through influence from the other language. For example, *aseguranza* is often used in the US to refer to medical insurance, but in monolingual contexts it means *safety*. The formal term for medical insurance would be *seguro médico*. Because Dr. Ortiz is a bilingual speaker and has transcultural competence, he knows both terms, but Spanish-language students may not be taught *aseguranza*, or may be taught that it is wrong.

The concept of translanguaging has origins in education research, and most research on the topic has been devoted to improving educators' understanding of language learners' speech and their approaches to it in the classroom (Nightingale and Safont 2019; Poza 2019) as well as teachers' own speech in language-learning classrooms (Musanti and Rodríguez 2017; Palmer et al. 2014). However, it has been usefully applied to global mental health initiatives (Andrews et al. 2018); for instance, Ortega and Prada (2020) found that practitioners who understand translanguaging are better able to provide patient-centered care. This chapter is the first use of a translanguaging lens to analyze doctor–patient interactions, however, and offers a deeper understanding than past research of the reasons why patients translanguage in health care settings and what types of language accommodations a doctor with transcultural competency makes. Dr. Ortiz's use of translanguaging practices in his interactions with patients, as this chapter describes, creates a space where patients can use their total speech repertoire. This in turn fosters *confianza*.[1]

Use of Loanwords and Semantic Extension

In some cases loanwords are needed to convey something specific. In example 1, Dr. Ortiz uses both the formal Spanish term and the loanword:

1) Loanword
Dr. Ortiz: *¿Y tiene incapacidad, desabilite?*
             Do you have disability?
Maribel (#10): *Sí.*
             Yes.

Incapacidad connotes a physical condition; the loanword *desabilite* invokes government support for people who have an *incapacidad*. It is needed because there is no equivalent word in Spanish that is not a loanword.

Semantic extension is more about conveying an informal tone and building *confianza* than conveying meaning. It primarily appears because it is part of patients' dialect, as illustrated when Teresa (early fifties, #16) uses *aseguranza*:

2) Semantic extension
Teresa: *Para ver si califico para alguna **aseguranza** para que me mande*
       con el cardiólogo
       To see if I qualify for any insurance to send me to the cardiologist

Like loanwords, terms or phrases with semantic extension are considered nonstandard, excluded from textbooks, and subject to correction in Spanish-language classrooms. This approach fails to prepare learners for the realities of language use in bilingual contexts. While Spanish learners need to know formal Spanish terms, it is also crucial that they know their local communities' colloquial uses and become aware of language attitudes in order to avoid stigmatizing people and their language varieties. Given that the language practices of Latino/as are diverse, teachers of medical Spanish should teach stu-

---

1. The approach in the literature on the pragmatic reasons for translanguaging (Musanti and Rodríguez 2017; Palmer et al. 2014; Poza 2019) and the sociolinguistics literature on code-switching (Jacobson 1982; Valdés 1982; Zentella 1997) informed my analysis of the interviews.

dents about the pragmatic or situational factors that affect these practices, including country of origin, region, dialect, socioeconomic status/education, and range of abilities in English, Spanish, or another language (e.g., an indigenous language), and promote the idea that there is a continuum of possibilities and that situational appropriateness is important.

Code-Switching as a Register

While all interviews include some loanwords from English, in four of the interviews there is extensive language-switching because the patients are bilingual. Many bilinguals in the US use code-switching to identify themselves as multicultural and as not fully assimilated Americans (Zentella 1997). Code-switching is prevalent among bilinguals in informal situations (Zentella 1997) and often perceived as an act of solidarity (Magaña 2016; Poza 2019). Bilinguals may perceive speaking only Spanish in an informal situation as "showing-off" because it may imply privileged access to education in Spanish or travel, whereas failing to use any Spanish when speaking to bilinguals may seem like an act of erasure (Elías-Olivares 1976; Magaña 2016; Vickers et al. 2015). Thus, code-switching offers a compromise (Valdés 1988).

Among bilingual speakers such as Dr. Ortiz and four of the patients whose interviews are studied here, code-switching can be a linguistically strategic choice as well as a socially productive one. Two languages present a greater number of language choices. Thus, switching languages involves drawing on greater linguistic resources. As Valdés points out, this richness is more than additive; she compared code-switching to playing a twelve-string guitar rather than using two six-stringed ones (1988, 126).

However, the general population widely misunderstands code-switching and refers to translanguaging practices between English and Spanish as Spanglish. When the Royal Spanish Academy first introduced Spanglish into its dictionary (2014), it defined it as follows:

*Modalidad del habla de algunos grupos hispanos de los Estados Unidos, en la que se mezclan, **deformándolos,** elementos léxicos y gramaticales del español y del inglés.*

Modality of speaking of some groups of Hispanics in the US, in which they mix lexical and grammatical elements of Spanish and English, **deforming** them.

In fact, three decades of literature has shown that code-switching reflects linguistic dexterity, follows certain grammatical rules, and is used stylistically and strategically (Poplack 1982; Toribio 2000; Zentella 1997). Although the Academy removed the term *deformándolos* shortly after at the request of sociolinguists, news sources, blogs, dictionaries, and social media posts continue to describe code-switching in stigmatized terms. For example, Angermeyer (2010) found that court interpreters in English-language courtrooms will rebuke claimants they are interpreting if they use any English, even a single word, saying that they should stay with the non-English language. While this was in part a consequence of interpreters believing that claimants were questioning the interpreter's competence to translate appropriately, they also upheld negative ideologies of code-switching as reflecting an inability to find the appropriate translation equivalent in English. But Zentella's (1997) groundbreaking ethnographic study on Puerto Rican bilinguals found that people who used English words while speaking Spanish also used the Spanish term, thus proving they knew the word in both languages. They may have failed to retrieve one or the other at a particular time, but they also may have code-switched for a social or pragmatic effect.

Sociolinguistics and applied linguistics research shows that switching languages has significant social and pragmatic purposes. Different studies have proposed different typologies, but there are noteworthy similarities among them. Gumperz's (1982) classifications have been particularly influential. Gumperz found that code-switching functioned for quotation, addressee specification, interjection, repetition, message qualification (where speakers separate statements from commentary), and personification versus objectivities (where speakers contrast their personal viewpoints with objective ones). Subsequent research on Spanish–English language alternation in the US revealed even longer lists (Jacobson 1982; Valdés 1982; Zentella 1997). Much of the research on code-switching has focused on in-group and informal interactions, even though code-switching occurs in institutional contexts as well, and formal contexts may be of particularly high stakes (Angermeyer 2010). As Altarriba and Santiago-Rivera (1994) suggest, medical patients may be willing to share more in one language than in the other and should be encouraged to switch languages, since this practice may support better medical outcomes.

The four bilingual patients in this study (Guadalupe, #3; Alejandro, #6; Ramón, #13; Cesar, #22) exhibited code-switching 234 times in total across their interviews. All their interviews were primarily in Spanish. As table 8 shows, patients contribute to the majority of code-switches: the doctor code-switches 43 times, or 18 percent of the time, and patients switch 191 times,

TABLE 8. Total code-switches by doctor and patients

PERSON	RAW NUMBER	PERCENTAGE	PER 1,000 WORDS
Doctor	43	18	1.8
Patients	191	82	3.3
Total	234	N/A	N/A

TABLE 9. Code-switching categories used by doctor and patients

PERSON	CONTEXTUAL	ELABORATION/ DEFINITION	CHECKING/ TAGS	EMPHASIS	QUOTATION
Doctor % out of 43	88	12	0	0	0
Patients % out of 191	71	6	17	3	3

or 82 percent of the time. Although this is partly because patients talk more than the doctor, when considering the rate of code-switches per 1,000 words, patients still switch at higher rates: 3.3 times per 1,000 words, while the doctor switches 1.8 times per 1,000 words.

The types of code-switches the patients and the doctor used differ slightly, as shown in table 9, but in both cases the contextual category dominates. This refers to switches influenced by a connection between the other language and the context or topic. Within the contextual category, patients often code-switch when using medical terms, whereas the doctor uses more triggered switches—that is, he code-switches because the patients do. Patients also code-switch for checking and tags (as discourse markers), for adding emphasis, and for quoting others. The doctor code-switches for elaboration or to offer a definition more often than patients do. These uses are explained with further examples and observations about their linguistic realizations in the following sections.

Contextual Code-Switching

Contextual code-switching, also called domain or topic shifts, overlaps with numerous other code-switching typologies and categorizations (Jacobson 1982). The connection between the other language and the context or topic may exist primarily in the mind of the speaker (Valdés 1982). For example, participants in Jacobson's (1982) study switched to Spanish to discuss home, family, and church; they switched to English to discuss employment, school, and business.

For Guadalupe, Alejandro, Ramón, and Cesar, medical terms tend to prompt language switches. Bilingual patients often enact this translanguaging practice when introducing medical terms or for names of organs, including *brain surgery, pancreas, gallbladder, cancer, kidneys, panic attack, anxiety,* and *cold sweat.* While switching often does not reflect a lack of knowledge of the terms in a particular language, it is possible that the four bilingual patients are not fluent in medical Spanish. However, they are fluent in conversational Spanish. It is also likely that, much like Jacobson's respondents in talking about work, they switch because they associate medical subjects with English, perhaps because English dominates in hospitals and clinics in the US.

In an example of the triggered switch, when Ramón code-switches by using the English term *brain surgery* to discuss a childhood accident, the doctor signals his understanding by replying "*¿Te hicieron* brain surgery?" "Did you have brain surgery?" This reflects the doctor's sociolinguistic awareness. If the doctor had answered using the Spanish term (*cirugía cerebral*), an implicit correction, Ramón might have interpreted it as an indicator of social distance due to different levels of access to education in Spanish. Although the doctor was socialized in Mexico, a monolingual Spanish-speaking country, and is an expert in medical registers of Spanish, the patient, thirty-five, although also Mexican American, was brought up in the US with two languages and is not as fluent in technical registers of Spanish as the doctor. Therefore, using *cirugía cerebral* would have indexed the doctor's high level of education in Spanish. By employing the patient's term *brain surgery,* the doctor demonstrates solidarity based on understanding both languages and cultures. Through his switch he tries to negotiate a change in the expected social distance between him and the patient, in this case decreasing that distance.

Guadalupe, a Mexican American female patient in her sixties, also prompts Dr. Ortiz to make a triggered switch:

3) Medical term and triggered switches
Dr. Ortiz: *En el setenta y cuatro le quitaron la—*
               In 1974 they removed the—
Guadalupe: *La* **gallbladder.**
               The gallbladder.
Dr. Ortiz: *La* **gallbladder.**
               The gallbladder.

Guadalupe: *Sí y luego empecé con* **pancreas attacks,** *malos y estuve aquí. Una de las veces, me dijeron que estaba muy mal y me metieron al hospital, un doctor, Fulano.*

Yes, and then I started getting pancreas attacks, bad ones, and I was here [at this facility]. During one of my visits, they said I was really ill and they hospitalized me, a doctor, John Doe [recommended it].

In this instance, the doctor is confirming a detail about Guadalupe's medical history: Guadalupe's 1974 surgical procedure to remove her gallbladder. Dr. Ortiz pauses to seek the Spanish terminology (*vesícula biliar*), but Guadalupe interrupts and offers the information "*la* gallbladder" with a feminine article. The doctor repeats the information to confirm with the patient, executing the triggered code-switch.

Dr. Ortiz follows Guadalupe for a longer switch in the next case:

Guadalupe: *Ahora que murió mi hijo, no muy bien pero antes—cuando me quitaron la* **kidney** *que salí ahí, le dije al* Doctor Peter, *¿ahora qué hago? Me dice,* "go home and live."

Since my son died, not so well but before—when they removed my kidney, after leaving [the facility], I told Doctor Peter, "now what do I do?" He says to me, "go home and live."

Dr. Ortiz: *¿Cuál* **kidney** *le quitaron?*

Which kidney did they remove?

Guadalupe: **The right side.**

Dr. Ortiz: **The right kidney?**

Guadalupe: **The right kidney.** *Lo perdí. Tenía un* **mass,** *un tumor de* **sixty-three millimeters.** *Fui y me sacó y que tenía cáncer. Era cáncer. Me dijo que la iba a sacar toda. Mi cáncer que me pegó en el* **pancreas** *era* **kidney cancer.** *Pero yo vivo mi vida.*

The right kidney. I lost it. I had a mass, a tumor that was sixty-three millimeters. I went [to the hospital] and it turned out I had cancer. It was cancer. He said he was going to remove the whole thing. The cancer that had developed in the pancreas was kidney cancer. But I go on with my life.

This longer triggered switch communicates that the doctor does not hold a stigmatized view of code-switching. It also prevents any disruption of the flow of the interview even if the patient does not know the term she uses in English in Spanish. Finally, it helps to create *confianza*. By using triggered switches, Dr. Ortiz signals that translanguaging is appropriate in that context and acknowledges its utility for obtaining a full medical history.

Another subcategory of contextual switches can occur when an equivalent in the other language does not exist, for example, *friolento/a* (i.e., someone with a tendency to be cold), and, as in the following example, feeling up or high. In a routine question during the twenty-question diagnostic for psychiatric disorders, toward the end of the interview, the doctor code-switches to ask whether patients felt "up" or "high." The English-language version question from the DSM-IV is, "Have you ever had a period of time when you were feeling '**up**' or '**high**' or 'hyper' or so **full** of energy or **full** of yourself that you got into trouble, or that other people thought you were not your usual self?"

The literature reports that English-speakers often use metaphors to describe feelings, such as describing happiness/euphoria as "up," and sadness/depression as "down" (Charteris-Black 2012; McMullen and Conway 2002). The literal translation of "feeling up/high" is *sentirse subido*, but it means having an inflated ego (Magaña 2019). For this reason the doctor routinely code-switches into English with all patients when he asks this question, as he seeks information about mania—an experience in which euphoria caused problems. This switch is necessary because the direct translation would convey the wrong meaning, but several patients, including a bilingual one, misunderstand the question, which disrupts the flow of the diagnostic section. In his question, the doctor uses both "up" and "high" to increase clarity; however, the question still causes confusion. In the following example, either the metaphorical use of euphoria as a vertical orientation (as implied in both "up" and "high"), the code-switch into English, or both confuse a bilingual patient.

4) Contextual (other)

Dr. Ortiz: *¿Has tenido una vez un periodo en tu vida donde estuvieras muy* **up,** *muy* **high,** *muy lleno de energía y que tuvieras dificultades con otras personas?*
Has there been a period in your life when you felt very up, very high, very full of energy and that it led you to have difficulties with other people?

Ramón: *No.*

Dr. Ortiz: *Y, ¿has estado muy enojado durante varios días y con pleitos con gente fuera de tu familia?*
And have you ever felt very angry for several days, or had fights/disagreements with people outside your family?

Ramón: *Sí.* [nods]
Yes.

Dr. Ortiz:	*Y como, ¿por qué?*
	And like, why?
Ramón:	*Pus, se me hace, me peleo cuando tomaba.*
	Well, I think, I fight when I would drink.
Dr. Ortiz:	*Ah, cuando tomabas.*
	Oh, when you would drink.
Ramón:	*Y les decía malas palabras.*
	And I would say bad words to them.
Dr. Ortiz:	*Si no tomas, ¿no?*
	If you don't drink, you don't?
Ramón:	*No* [giggles]

Ramón had said earlier, "*hablo cosas que no debo hablar; luego me arrepiento*" (I say things I shouldn't say; then later I regret it), which suggests he may have experienced mania, as do some of his answers after he responds to the question about feeling "up" or "high" that contains the code-switch. Thus, his "no" regarding feeling "up" or "high" likely reflects confusion (Magaña 2019).

Patients who are not bilingual find this question confusing. Martín (early fifties, #17) changes his answer from yes to no after the doctor clarifies that the question refers to getting into trouble. It is consequently not clear whether Martín understands the metaphor or the code-switch. Miguel (mid-forties, #7) also changes his answer, in his case, from no to yes. Ultimately, code-switching doesn't entirely make the sentence accessible to patients. Although Dr. Ortiz has experience working with rural Mexican communities in Mexico and does not have trouble understanding patients' metaphorical conceptualizations of mental health symptoms and diseases, he may have overestimated how much the English language (and its metaphors) affects people's understanding of mental health. However, as his interactions with Martín and Miguel suggest, he is able to repair the breakdown in communication that the metaphor caused by discussing the question of problematic euphoria further.

Using English because a specific phrase does not have an equivalent in Spanish is another contextual type of code-switching. (While similar to loan-words, these instances qualify as code-switching because the word has not been assimilated into Spanish.) For example, with Alejandro (#6), a male patient in his early thirties, using the common English phrase *out of the blue* keeps conversation smooth:

6) Contextual (other)

| Dr. Ortiz: | *Los ataques de pánico que tienes, ¿son en alguna situación en especial?* |

The panic attacks that you get, do you get them in certain situations?

Alejandro: *Son en veces nomás en formas en que—¿Qué es lo que voy a hacer,* **you know?** *¿Qué es lo que va a ser,* **my future, you know?** *¿Qué es lo que pienso y en veces—si he hecho unas cosas en mi vida que—como ahorita no tengo licencia para manejar porque por problemas que he tenido hace un año. Entonces eso para mí—en veces pienso en eso y me pongo* **panic** *porque digo,* **how am I gonna get around?** *¿Cómo voy a llegar [**inaudible**] a trabajar? Pero yo, luego pienso y tengo que calmarme porque si no se va a hacer peor.*

They only happen sometimes in ways that—What am I going to do, you know? What will be of my future, you know. What am I thinking and sometimes—Yes, I have done things in my life that—like right now I don't have a driver's license because of problems I had a year ago. So that for me—sometimes I think about that and I panic because I'm like, how am I going to get around? How am I going to get to work? [Alejandro works in construction.] But then I think, and I have to calm down because if not it could get worse.

Dr. Ortiz: *OK. ¿Y pueden salir así* **out of the blue** *también?*

OK. Do they also happen like out of the blue?

Alejandro: **Yeah, yeah. Out of the blue, they just—like Sat—***el domingo.*

Yeah, yeah. Out of the blue, they just—like Sat—on Sunday.

Dr. Ortiz's code-switch is also triggered, in that it follows a number of switches in Alejandro's speech. We can speculate that Dr. Ortiz notes the patient's comfort in switching languages throughout the interaction before employing this code-switch. Interestingly, Alejandro repeats the doctor's phrase when he answers "Yeah, yeah. Out of the blue." He could have answered the question affirmatively without repeating the phrase, but he articulates alignment and solidarity with the doctor by repetition instead. Here the patient's switch indexes his acceptance of the doctor's bilingual membership.

Elaboration/Definition

Code-switching for elaboration or definition occurs when the speaker switches languages in order to add information or details about the topic of interaction (Magaña 2018b). For instance, in example 7, Alejandro begins explaining a difficult point in his life in Spanish and then switches momentarily to English to add more information about how he felt. Alejandro admits to his doctor that there was a time where he felt he made bad choices (*Iba por muy mal camino*). He then switches to English, an elaboration switch, to add additional details about how he felt (saying I'd forget about myself) and then switches back to Spanish, the main language of the interaction:

7) Elaboration / definition

Alejandro: *Iba por muy mal camino.* **I'd forget about myself.** *Y entonces. . . .*
I was going down the wrong path. I'd forget about myself. And then. . . .

The doctor uses this code-switch type strategically to make sure patients understand key medical terms or phrases. In the next example, he uses this strategy for the phrase *panic attacks* during a consultation with Cesar (#22), a Mexican American patient in his mid-thirties. The following excerpt (8) exemplifies how he uses this type of switch as a definition, which also functions as an intentional teaching moment:

8) Elaboration / definition

Dr. Ortiz: *¿ Entonces cuáles son los síntomas iniciales?*
So what are the initial symptoms?

Cesar: *Los síntomas que siento; siento que se me, cuando me empiezan a dar los, los, la **anxiety**; empiezo a sentir como la garganta seca. Empiezo a sentir como que se me va el aire. Hay veces que, bueno, ahorita ya últimamente no, pero anteriormente dos veces sentía como que las piernas se me dormían y como que me quería, así como desmayar.*
The symptoms that I have; I feel that it's, when I start to get the, the, the anxiety; I start to feel like my throat is dry. I start to feel like out of air. There are times when, well, not really recently, but twice before I've feel like my legs would get numb and like I wanted to, like faint.

Dr. Ortiz: Mhm

Cesar: *Sentía así como que el aire no . . . y sentía . . . Había veces que sentía como que quería arrancarme la camisa.*
I felt like the air was not . . . And I felt . . . There were times that I felt like I wanted to rip off my shirt.

Dr. Ortiz: *Aja.*
Aha.

Cesar: ¿OK? Y como brincar de la ventana.
            OK? And like jump out the window.

Dr. Ortiz: ¿Y el corazón así? [Taps his chest multiple times]
            And your heart [beats] like this?

Cesar: Yeah. Y, este, llegó a un punto que me hice a un lado del camino
            como queriendo vomitar, pero no podía vomitar, solo augh . . .
            Yeah. And, well, it got to the point that I pulled over to the side
            of the road like wanting to vomit, but I couldn't, just augh.

Dr. Ortiz: Nauseas.
            Nausea.

Cesar: Yeah. Nauseas y hasta que fui al hospital y me dieron una pastilla.
            Yeah. Nausea and [it happened] until I went to the hospital and
            they gave me a pill.

Dr. Ortiz: ¿Sudor?
            Any sweating?

Cesar: Sí, cold sweat.
            Yes, cold sweat.

Dr. Ortiz: Se llaman ataques de pánico.
            They're called panic attacks.

Cesar: Oh, ¿eso es lo que es?
            Oh, is that what it is?

Dr. Ortiz: Mhm. Panic attacks.

Here, the doctor switches to English to add clarity to his definition of panic attacks. As above, he switches to English after Cesar has made several switches. Thus, the doctor indexes a bilingual membership and solidarity.

Checking and Tags

Bilinguals often use checking and tags (e.g., "right?" or "you know?") to seek the listener's opinion or approval or use general discourse markers ("yeah," "so") as continuers when telling their stories. The doctor only uses discourse markers in Spanish such as ¿no? ¿sí? and ¿verdad?, mostly as checking devices. He also uses okay, a loanword often used in Mexican Spanish. However, a couple of the patients uses tags in English, such as in example (6) above where Alejandro says "you know" and "yeah" in English. Cesar (#22) inserts "you know?" as he tells the doctor that he does not understand the source of his depression:

9) Checking and tags

Cesar: *Y pues no, no sé qué es lo que esté ocasionando. Toda mi vida he andado,* **you know,** *alrededor de personas y nunca me he sentido así, y últimamente . . .*

And well, no, I do not know what is causing this. All my life I have been, you know, around people and I've never felt like this, and lately . . .

10) Checking and tags

Cesar: *Mis papás eran de las personas que no los sacaban. Muy pocas veces los llevaban a las tiendas. Este,* **so,** *estábamos muy tapados.*
My parents were of the people who did not take us out. There were very few times when they took us to the stores. Well, so, we were, very sheltered.

Dr. Ortiz does not respond in kind, possibly because these discourse markers are not part of his bilingual repertoire. Dr. Ortiz received bilingual education in Mexico and is fluent in written and spoken English, but at the time of the interviews, he had only been living in the US for five years. Employing discourse markers can signal advanced proficiency in a second language; compared with native speakers, second-language learners of English have more limited uses of discourse (Fung and Carter 2007).

Emphasis

Bilinguals may switch languages for emphasis to draw special attention to something they have uttered. Repeating a word in the other language adds emphasis, as in this example with Alejandro:

11) Emphasis

Dr. Ortiz: *La agresión de tu padre, ¿te regresa de repente? ¿Tienes* **flashbacks?**
Does your father's aggression suddenly come back to you? Do you get flashbacks?

Alejandro: No.

Dr. Ortiz: *¿[Tienes] pesadillas?*
Any nightmares?)

Alejandro: **Before**—*antes sí.*
Before, before yes I did.

In line with Zentella's (1997) research, the code-switching does not reflect any difficulty recalling the term in the other language. Alejandro uses it to empha-size that he no longer has nightmares, although he did once.

Quotation

Code-switching also occurs when a bilingual speaker directly or indirectly quotes someone. As we see in example (12) from the medical history portion of Guadalupe's interview, she strategically code-switches to separate the quote from her own discourse when quoting her surgeon.

12) Emphasis
Guadalupe: *Le dije [al doctor]* **"do it."** *Y me dijo,* **"I like the way you think."**
I told the doctor "do it." And he said to me, "I like the way you think."

As Zentella (1997) pointed out, such quotes might not use the language of the original quotation (94). Since it can be difficult in spoken discourse to distin-guish direct quotations from their surroundings, marking the statement in this way is a useful linguistic tool. The nonjudgmental bilingual context that doctor and patients create in these interviews may have invited Guadalupe to switch to English to clarify the punctuation of her sentence.

Conclusions

A common misconception about code-switching is that it is due to lexical gaps in one language. Although this may be the case for some of the patients in this study, it is clear that the interlocutors used code-switching for contex-tual reasons. Bilingual patients often switch to English for medical terms and other terms/phrases they associate with an English-language context. Patients also strategically used code-switching for emphasis and for quoting others.

Dr. Ortiz code-switches in this medical context as a discourse strategy to connect with bilingual patients. In doing so, he creates a space for translan-guaging "between linguistic structures, systems, and modalities, and going beyond them," and "integrate[d] social spaces (and thus 'language codes') that have formerly been practiced separately in different places" (García and Wei 2014, 24). The effect is articulating solidarity; he understands his patients' situation as bilingual/bicultural people in the US, even though he had been living in the US for less than five years at the time of the interviews. He also shows affective involvement, since code-switching is an intimate register of speaking that is reserved for in-group use and can be stigmatized. Therefore, code-switches mark the doctor's embrace of the in-group, accommodation of his patients' preferred register, and sociolinguistic awareness of bilingual norms in the US.

By using colloquialisms as illustrated in the preceding chapter and translanguaging in this chapter, the doctor demonstrates his acceptance of his patients' varieties. As Martínez (2011) points out, public health workers have framed measures to broach language barriers as "language assistance," but acceptance of a patient's language needs is far more likely to produce effective results—such as, in this case, building a temporary connection between doctor and patient that facilitates patient care. Dr. Ortiz demonstrates language acceptance through his sociolinguistic awareness of the language varieties of Latino/as in the US, a descriptive view of and attitude toward language varieties, and the ability to accommodate to the variety of patients in order not to mark, even subconsciously, inferiority/superiority distinctions between varieties.

Dr. Ortiz's sociolinguistic awareness allows him to provide his patients transculturally competent health care. By engaging in translanguaging practices with patients, he tries to create a trustworthy environment for them, which relates directly to the cultural construct of *confianza*. Creating *confianza* specifically by embracing bilingual practices is essential in this context; research shows that patients may be willing to share more embarrassing information or may be better equipped to express their concerns in one language over the other (Santiago-Rivera and Altarriba 2002). Dr. Ortiz encourages patients to express themselves using all their linguistic resources in this sensitive context of psychiatric interviews by creating a space for translanguaging.

Successfully creating space for translanguaging practices requires providers to know the linguistic practices of the communities they serve, as Latino/as in the US are a diverse group with a range of languages or language-variety uses. The provider adjusts his interactions accordingly and code-switches with the four bilingual speakers in the sample, since code-switching with monolingual Spanish speakers in the medical context can be a disempowering experience for the patient (Vickers et al. 2015). A medical provider and leader in the field of medical Spanish, Dr. Pilar Ortega, calls for the inclusion of translanguaging in doctor training, explaining that such curricula should "acknowledg[e] how local populations use their linguistic repertoires in the medical context" (Ortega and Prada 2020, 252–53).

Dr. Ortiz's awareness of the linguistic practices of his patients in rural California and of transcultural competency makes his adaptation possible.

His performance of his local knowledge in specific situations helps create the interpersonal bonds that are likely to be conducive to high-quality patient-centered care. These performances are illustrated in different examples throughout this book, where the doctor displays *personalismo, simpatía* (as described in chapters 2 and 3), *confianza* (this chapter), and *respeto.*

Chapter 6 complements the findings reported here by focusing on grammatical analysis of interpersonal language and describing Dr. Ortiz's display of *respeto.* The grammatical analysis in that chapter reveals the specific components of the language used in the interviews, particularly the linguistic strategies they use to make meaning in a transcultural context. The analysis illustrates how each interlocutor indexes his or her social role and the ways in which *respeto* is conveyed at the language level.

Insights for Medical Practitioners and Interpreters

- This chapter highlighted code-switching, a bilingual practice common in the US, and revealed that code-switching has a distinct function for both Dr. Ortiz and his patients. Bilingual patients use it often for contextual reasons, including switching to English for medical terms. The doctor switches languages as a way to close the social distance, to display solidarity, and as a teaching tool, for definitions and clarity.
- It is essential for providers to know about the language background of Latino/as who make up significant numbers of their patients. Translanguaging practices, like code-switching, convey much about the speaker's social identity, ideologies, and culture. For bilinguals, code-switching may be sociopolitically charged. They have typically faced negative attitudes from those who misunderstand code-switching and stigmatize it, but for some bilinguals who recognize it as a tool they use with particular ease, it may be a source of pride. When patients use these translanguaging practices and a medical practitioner responds in kind, it may support trust.
- Engaging in translanguaging practices such as code-switching can be an intimate way to communicate solidarity and *confianza* (trust) with someone. Creating trust is particularly crucial in psychiatric interviews; therefore, providers should be knowledgeable about how bilinguals in the US speak and embrace this use. Creating space for translanguaging with patients indicates skill in transcultural competence.
- In medical Spanish classrooms it is essential to incorporate lessons in sociolinguistic awareness with respect to translanguaging practices

(code-switching, loanwords, other English-language influences). These phenomena occur naturally when languages are in contact. In fact, the most fluent bilinguals can code-switch, and they do so for linguistically strategic reasons. Instructors should educate language learners about translanguaging research since misunderstanding bilingual language practices could be damaging.

CHAPTER 6

Expressing Verbal Modality
and Other Politeness Strategies
in Psychiatric Interviews

THE GOAL OF THIS CHAPTER is to discuss how an interpersonal relationship between Dr. Ortiz and his patients unfolds linguistically during their interactions and how they express politeness. While the preceding chapters described more abstract levels of register and genre, this chapter reports on an analysis of the interviews at the most concrete level of language. It details the interpersonal language choices the doctor makes in seeking patient information and reveals concrete examples of how Dr. Ortiz shows *respeto* (deferential behavior based on age, gender, and social position of interlocutor) and, as a result, transcultural competence. A focus on politeness and interpersonal language is useful for this study because it offers specific tools for studying the relationships between interlocutors during an interaction. As linguist health communication and systemic functional linguistics (SFL) expert Suzanne Eggins explains, "Dialogue is the means language gives us for expressing interpersonal meanings about roles and attitudes. Being able to take part in dialogue, then, means being able to negotiate the exchange of interpersonal meanings [and] being able to realize social relationships with other language users" (2004, 144). In this chapter I turn to two critical features of politeness: mitigation (specifically, verbal modality) and alignment (specifically, posing biased questions).

Mitigation and Verbal Modality

Research shows that mitigation is a concept central to interpersonal meaning in medical discourse (Caffi 2007; Figueras Bates 2020; Flores-Ferrán 2010, 2012; Magaña 2017). Mitigation is an essential linguistic resource in that it enables speakers to both reach their discursive aims and negotiate interpersonal distances (Caffi 2007). When people mitigate a statement, it helps them avoid unnecessary risks, responsibilities, and conflicts (Caffi 2007, 3). Speakers can use a range of mitigation devices, including hedges and verbal modality. In medical interactions mitigation is a part of politeness strategies and a tool for negotiating social and power roles and cultural expectations and values (Caffi 1999; Cordella 2007; Delbene 2004; Flores-Ferrán 2010, 2012). In her case study of client and therapist interactions, Flores-Ferrán (2010) proposes the following mitigating devices:

Modal verbs: *creo* "I think"/ *supongo* "I suppose"/ *me imagino* "I imagine"
Hedge: *más o menos* "more or less"/ *tal como* "such as"
Bushes: *como* "like" (approximator)
Shield: *uno* "one" (generalization as opposed to pointing out a specific person)
Time deixis: conditional, subjunctive
Redundant verb clauses: repeating has a downgrade effect in this case
Tag questions: *¿cierto?* "right?"

Studies on mitigation can offer insights about the issues patients face in medical interactions. For instance, a study on the conversation of doctors and seropositive patients in Uruguay reveals that mitigation is a common discourse strategy when discussing HIV, a taboo and sensitive subject (Delbene 2004).

Throughout their interactions, doctor and patients in this study negotiate their social roles and mediate their power differences as revealed through analysis of mitigation and, specifically, verbal modality, the linguistic choices speakers make to communicate probability, the degree to which something is probable. Modality devices are multifunctional since people use them to express hesitation, solidarity, politeness, respect, and/or humility, all of which are important in negotiating an interpersonal relationship (Hyland 1996). Mitigation studies within pragmatics make a crucial contribution to our understanding of verbal modality in SFL. These theoretical approaches are complementary. Pragmatics research has offered essential contributions regarding oral discourse, whereas SFL has predominantly been developed using written language but offers rich resources for grammatical analysis. In my study on verbal modality in medical interviews, I reported on their frequency and the grammar of modality devices from an SFL perspective (Magaña 2017). In this chapter I focus on the multiple functions of verbal modality and introduce other politeness strategies. In conclusion, I explain how these politeness strategies are relevant to discussions of transcultural competence in health interactions.

My quantification of the use of modality devices counts only those that expressed probability. In total there were 1,429 instances of verbal modality in the twenty-three interviews. Patients tend to use more modality devices than the doctor; the circumstances in which each uses verbal modality differ, as does the preference type between patients and the doctor (Magaña 2017). The most common were modal verbs, bushes, and tags. The following sections explain each of these categories and demonstrate their use and functions in the interviews. By focusing on verbal modality, I also uncover information about how speakers negotiate their social roles in the psychiatric interview genre.

Modal Verbs

Using modal verbs (e.g., *Pienso que* "I think that") is a common way to express probability in oral contexts. In example 1 below, taken from an interaction with Roberto, a male patient in his forties (#8), the patient uses the modal verb *creer*, to believe. This is the patient's response when the doctor asks him about his chief complaint, the reason for the referral to the psychiatric interview:

1) Modal verb
Roberto: **Creo que** *tengo la enfermedad mentalmente.*
           I believe my illness is mental.

The most commonly used modal verbs and phrases in the interviews are *creo que* (I believe), *pienso* (I think), *puede que* (it could be that), *me parece que* (it seems to me that), and *se me hace que* (it seems to me that). These modal verbs can be placed before or after a statement or a response, as illustrated in example 2, a patient's response to Dr. Ortiz asking her during the medical history section of the interview whether she takes any drugs (meaning recreational drugs), a question he asks of all patients:

2) Modal verb
Amalia: *No, de ninguna,* **yo pienso.**
          No, not of any kind, **I think.**

Amalia (#20) says that she is not using any drugs that she is aware of, but then she creates space for ambiguity by adding *"yo pienso."* By this point in the interview, the patient has admitted that she has been feeling depressed. She feels disconnected from her husband and her fifteen grown children. Because of her various health problems, Amalia takes eight types of medication to treat diabetes, anxiety, and insomnia. She adds that when she feels frustrated, she takes more medication than prescribed and that her general practitioner has expressed concerns over her dependence on medication. Thus, the modal verb adds room for alternative interpretations of the classification of "drug use" and displaces responsibility from her answer. On the patient's end, modality invites her to add important information about her medical history (her potential prescription overuse) after making the denial.

Se me hace (it seems to me) and *supongo que* (I suppose that) are also in the modal verb category. Speakers used *se me hace* more often than *supongo que*. This example, with a patient, Norma (female, mid-forties, #12) who has diabetes and chronic pain, concerns blood sugar levels:

3) Modal verbs

Dr. Ortiz: *¿Cuánto tenía; no le dijo?*
What was your level; did he not tell you?

Norma: *Me dijo que, **se me hace que** cien de setentaiuno. Pero me dijo, **a la mejor** en el futuro **puede ser más.** Pues sí, porque ahorita me dio unas hojas para yo tomar como lectura, ¿verdad?*
He told me that, **it seems to me** that it was 100 over 70. But he told me, **maybe** in the future **it could be** more. Well, for now he gave me some sheets so that I could read them, you see?

Norma uses verbal modality to present medical information carefully, which is crucial here because she's reporting information that a third party relayed to her. As in the previous examples, by using a modal adjunct, the patient displaces responsibility from the reliability of her answer and positions herself as the nonexpert. Verbal modality, then, is a resource that patients use to index their social roles in this context.

The doctor also uses modal verbs but to a different effect, since they are directed at the patients. For instance, he asks Jazmín (female, late twenties, #15) whether she believes something occurred that triggered her depression. By this point in the interview, the patient has told the doctor that she has been feeling depressed (manifested in frequent crying and difficulty getting out of bed) and has had frequent headaches and sleeplessness for about a year. As she offers this information, the doctor mainly confirms her answers using continuers ("mhm hum") and then probes into more details with the following question.

4) Modal verbs

Dr. Ortiz: *¿Y tú qué **crees** que pasó hace un año que te empezaste a sentir deprimida?*

What is it that **you think** happened a year ago when you started feeling depressed?

By including this modal verb in his question, the doctor displaces responsibility from the patient and creates a more comfortable environment for the patient by inviting her to share her thoughts. The patient's response that she *thinks* her depression began when her son was born suggests that he succeeds. The doctor's use of the second-person singular pronoun *tú* (you) emphasizes the patient's centrality and reinforces the invitation. Caffi (1999) refers to this technique as "deresponsabilization," and she also finds that it recurs in her data analysis of doctor–patient interactions. By displacing responsibility from patients, the doctor is taking steps toward gaining their trust, which is crucial in a psychiatric interview.

Como (Like) as Bushes

In addition to modal verbs, doctor and patients use "bushes," words that make the propositional content "less precise" or "semantically fuzzy" (Caffi 1999). Both doctor and patients frequently used the prepositional item *como* (like) as a bush (as in Flores-Ferrán 2010, 2012; Caffi 1999).

Numerous research studies have been devoted to the multifunctional uses of "like" found across varieties of English (Mihatsch 2009; Tagliamonte 2005). However, little research has been conducted on *como* in Spanish spoken in the US. An exception, studying its use among Spanish-heritage language students in California, found that bilingual students use *como* in similar ways to American English "like" because of language-contact influence (Sánchez-Muñoz 2007). The patients in this study used *como* in a variety of ways, but not as semantically empty interjections like that found in the speech of young adults (Mihatsch 2009; Sánchez-Muñoz 2007). These differences are likely due to the particular sociodemographic profiles of the patients, as most patients are not bilingual and are adults. The most common use of *como* was as a bush, and the results here report on those uses.

Como (like) as a preposition can mean "similar to" and as a modality device has high probability. SFL considers "like" to be a "circumstantial element" that can function as a type of process participating in the relationship between a subject and complement or adjunct (Halliday and Matthiessen 2004). For instance, "like" functions as the relational processes (verb) "to be" and "to have" in certain contexts (Halliday and Matthiessen 2004). In the sentence "The disease is curable," the relational process ("is") attributes characteristics ("curable") to the entity ("the disease"). In other words, the attribute defines or describes the entity. Similarly, in the following example, the circumstantial element *como* attributes the characteristic *muy caliente* (very warm) to the entity (the sensor/subject)—in this case, the patient (female, early fifties, #16):

5) Bushes

Teresa: *Me empiezo a sentir **como** muy caliente.*
               I start feeling like very warm.

Patients commonly used bushes when explaining their symptoms and offering medical information. *Como* creates some ambiguity, and through its use, patients express some doubt. During the clinical history part of the interview, Teresa explains that she deals with numerous health problems: diabetes, cholesterol, and high blood pressure. She says, though, that lack of health insurance is a primary concern. After the doctor listens attentively to her narrative of both physiological symptoms and financial obstacles, he asks about her anxiety levels and collects information about panic attacks. Her response uses "*como*" frequently:

6) Bushes

Teresa: *En las noches, en las noches me palpita **como** taquicardias. Me*
               *pega mucha taquicardia y me empieza **como** . . . **como que** me*
               *empiezo a sentir **como** muy caliente, **como** sudando, **como** con*
               sudor y me empieza a dar mucha taquicardia.
               At night, at night, my heart beats **like** tachycardia. I get a lot
               of tachycardia and I start feeling **like** . . . **like** I start to feel **like**
               very warm, **like** I'm sweating, **like** I sweat and I start to get a lot
               of tachycardia.

By using *como* in explaining that she felt "like very warm, like I'm sweating," the patient signals that hot and sweaty are an approximation of her feelings. In this case *como* "like" is used to conceptualize the chosen expression modified as the target concept drawing on their similarities (Mihatsch 2009). The following examples further illustrate this strategy and how the doctor uses it to negotiate information from patients.

7) Bushes

Dr. Ortiz: *¿Cómo es la depresión? ¿**Como** tristeza o **como** vacío? ¿Cómo?*

	What is the depression like? Like sadness or like emptiness? How?
Érica (#20):	*Eh, yo no sé qué será vacío, pero yo siento **como** que mi estó-mago me brinca mucho y **como** que me tiembla. . . .*
	Um, I don't know what emptiness is like, but I feel that my stomach twitches and shakes. . . .
Dr. Ortiz:	Hmm [nods]
Érica:	*Mucho dolor de cabeza . . .*
	Very painful headaches
Dr. Ortiz:	Hmm [nods]
Érica:	*A veces me siento **como** bien aguados mis pies.*
	Sometimes I feel my legs are like jello.
Dr. Ortiz:	Hmm [nods], *¿**Como** débil?*
	Like weak?

The doctor uses *como* when posing some of his questions to allow patients to give an estimate of their answers, avoiding putting them on the spot. Frequently, when he asks about patients' height and weight, he uses *como*, as illustrated in the following example:

8) Bushes

Dr. Ortiz:	*¿**Como** cuánto mide?*
	About how tall are you?
María (#18):	*Uhm.*
Dr. Ortiz:	***Como** 3 por ahí, **como** 4.*
	About 3, or about 4.
María:	***Como** 4'11" **se me hace** o no me acuer[do]. . . .*
	About 4'11" it seems to me, I don't remem. . . .
Dr. Ortiz:	*¿4'11"?*
María:	***Parece.***
	It seems like it.

In creating space for ambiguity using *como*, the doctor makes a safe space for patients to answer even if their response is only an estimate. Thus, he reduces the risk of self-contradiction, or potential conflict (Caffi 1999). Example 8 reflects the success of this strategy. The patient responds with an estimate and again uses modality devices (*como, se me hace,* and *parece*). The doctor and patients also use *como* for clarification purposes. For instance, the speakers commonly use it to negotiate meaning by describing how they feel using a semantically similar item (Mihatsch 2009). The doctor uses these to offer tangible comparisons and mediate comprehension.

In the following example, the doctor and patient discuss Roberto's anxiety (early forties, #8). Roberto faces numerous stressors, including having an unstable, low-paid job that prevents him from sending financial help to his ill parents in Mexico. When the doctor asks for clarification of Roberto's symptoms, the doctor offers two specific choices for how he may be feeling to specify Roberto's symptoms further.

9) Bushes

Dr. Ortiz: *¿Es nada más falta de aire, **como que** no hay suficiente aire o siente **como que** se está ahogando?*
Is it just shortness of breath, like there is not enough air, or do you feel like you're suffocating.

Roberto: *Uhm . . . falta de aire.*
Uhm . . . shortness of breath.

Dr. Ortiz: *Falta de . . .*
Shortness of . . . [repeating to himself]

Roberto: ***Como que** siento desde debajo de aquí, del pecho. . . .*
It's like I feel it from below, from here, from my chest. . . .

Dr. Ortiz: ***¿Como que** no jala suficiente?*
Like it's not working properly?

Roberto: *Ahí.*
That.

Using bushes to negotiate meaning with patients allows the doctor to share medical knowledge while allowing patients to have a central role in offering health information about themselves. This is one way in which the doctor avoids invoking his social status.

Tags

Tags are linguistic devices that hedge the strength of a statement or question (Holmes 1986). As mitigating devices, these are also highly multifunctional (Flores-Ferrán 2010, 2012; Fraser 1980; Holmes 1986; Labov and Fanshel 1977). Patients and doctor use tags to indicate continuation (a polite form of signaling to the interlocutor that they have the floor), seek alignment (engaging the speaker to include her in the interaction), and express probability; this subsection reports specifically on tags that expressed possibility. The most commonly used tags in the study were "*¿no?*" "right?" "*¿sí?*" "yes?" and "*¿verdad?*" "right?"

The doctor uses tags frequently as confirmation checks, more often than patients do. The tags express uncertainty, seeking confirmation or correction from the patients. The following example stems from an interaction between Dr. Ortiz and Miguel (male, forties, #7), where the doctor shares information about how to obtain prescription glasses. Miguel asks whether he has to go to the doctor's office to obtain glasses.

10) Tags
Miguel: *Tengo que ir con un doctor, ¿no?*
            I have to go see a doctor, right?

The doctor strategically uses tags to confirm information from patients and mediate any uncertainty he has about their responses. This strategy is illustrated with Cesar (male, mid-thirties, #22), who deals with severe anxiety.

11) Tags
Dr. Ortiz: *¿Andas todo el día preocupado por algo?*
            Do you worry all day about something?
Cesar: *Yo diría que sí.*
            I would say yes.
Dr. Ortiz: *¿Sí?*
            Yes?
Cesar: *Sí, hay veces que sí, uhm . . .*
            Yes, there are times that I do, uhm . . .

Patients also use tags to confirm and negotiate information with the doctor. The example below is an excerpt from an interaction between the doctor and Roberto (#8), who also deals with anxiety and panic attacks. Toward the beginning of the interview, Roberto tells the doctor that, when stressed, he feels out of breath, "*me falta aire.*" He says that when he has an attack, he feels anxious and feels like his body is overheating and sweating. Toward the end of the interview, the doctor recycles the patients' words to probe further, asking what happens when he feels out of breath ("*que le falta aire*"). Roberto's response includes a tag:

12) Tags
Roberto: *O sea, en realidad no sé cómo explicar lo que siento, pero pues sí,*
            ¿verdad?
            I mean, the truth is I don't know how to explain how I feel, but
            yes, right?

The patient explains that he is unsure how to explain further what he feels and then uses the tag *¿verdad?* In this case the patient is confirming that the doctor understood the details he had offered about his episodes. The doctor replies, "OK," signaling that he has, in fact, understood, and moves on to his next question.

Although there are other means of realizing confirmation checks nonverbally (for instance, through gestures or even silence), tags are an important resource for achieving this negotiation of meaning by checking information and opening space for interpretation.

Biased Questions as Alignment Strategy

Asking biased questions is another interpersonal strategy the doctor uses. Biased questions imply an initial hypothesis with respect to the answer, as the following example illustrates.

13) Biased questions
Dr. Ortiz: *¿No tiene trabajo?*
             You don't work right now?[1]
Érica (#19): *No, horita no.*
             No, not right now.

Biased questions allow the doctor to align with patients as he confirms or obtains information from them without putting them on the spot. The doctor's question is biased in the sense that it implies that the patient does not work, unlike a formulation such as "do you work right now?"

The doctor's biased question in example 13 employs negative polarity. The choice to use negative polarity informs us about the transcultural knowledge of the doctor given that, among Mexican Spanish speakers, posing questions with negative polarity displays politeness (Curcó 1998; Garachana Camarero 2008).[2] The mere presence of negation is not sufficient for its classification

---

1. There are different ways to translate these questions into English using negative polarity. For instance, "*¿No tiene trabajo ahorita?*" can be translated as either "Don't you work right now?" or "You don't work right now?" The two forms have distinct connotations. The former seems judgmental and therefore is impolite, which would inaccurately describe the doctor's intention. The latter more accurately represents the doctor's intention: to be polite and to postulate a hypothesis about the answer.

2. For Spanish commands, Garachana Camarero (2008) explains that it is politer to pose a question with a negative particle, as in "*¿No tendrías un poco de sal para darme?*" "You wouldn't have some salt to give me, would you?" because the presence of the *no* attenuates the potential refusal. In her comparative study of Spanish speakers from Spain and Mexico, Curcó (1998) explains that in Mexican societies, reinforcement of a positive image is an important

as negative polarity, since "no" can be used to contradict or confirm a statement, or to function as a tag (Eggins and Slade 2005). Instead, the negation has to affect the whole polarity of the clause in order to be considered negative polarity.

Because the doctor asked most of the questions, the discussion of the following results focuses on how the doctor, not the patients, formulates questions. Of the 1,515 he asks across the interviews, 154 are biased questions.

The doctor uses these biased questions strategically. Some are posed with the negative particle "no" as well as those with the conjunction "*ni*" (nor) and adverbs that function as adjuncts to refer to time as "*nunca*" and "*jamás*" (both meaning "never"). The analysis reveals that the primary functions or biased questions are for confirming information, introducing a taboo topic, and establishing inclusivity. The following discussion presents each of these categories to illustrate how meaning-making is revealed when analyzing biased questions.

A primary function of biased interrogatives is to confirm patients' responses. The following example illustrates the grammatical resources the doctor employs to formulate biased interrogatives:

14) Biased questions

Dr. Ortiz: *¿Se llevan bien?*
                 Do you get along well [with your husband]?[3]

Jazmín (#15):   *Sí.* [Nodding].
                 Yes. [Nodding].

Dr. Ortiz: *¿No tienen problemas grandes?*
                 You don't have big problems?

Jazmín: *No.* [Shakes head].
                 No. [Shakes head].

Dr. Ortiz: *¿Los normales?*
                 Normal ones?

Jazmín: *¡Normales!* [Nodding]. *Problemas normales.*
                 Normal ones! [Nodding]. Normal problems.

---

value, far more so than in Spain. Thus, Mexicans find the interrogative with negation to be the politer form, but Spaniards make no such distinction (Curcó 1998).

3. The question is an example of alternative structures to form biased questions. The question is considered biased because the doctor is implying that the patient will answer affirmatively. Alternative versions of the question would be "*¿Se llevan mal?*" "Do you not get along?," where the inclination is toward negative polarity (hence also a biased question) and "*¿Cómo se llevan?*," where the question is neutral and unbiased. In a study where participants were mostly middle-class Mexicans, Koike found that "negation in Spanish and English suggestions and requests is not used to soften or mitigate the proposition" (1994, 525).

The bias in *¿No tienen problemas grandes?* "You don't have big problems?" reflects the preceding. Had he said instead "*¿Tienen problemas grandes?* Do you have big problems?" it would have implied that he disbelieved Jazmín's statement that she did get along with her husband. Therefore, the patient could have interpreted this hypothetical question as rude since the doctor would have been disregarding her previous answer. Instead, by using negative polarity, the doctor seeks to confirm the information in a more culturally appropriate manner and shows respect. The doctor asks Jazmín yet another question to once more confirm the patient's response: *¿Los normales?* "Normal ones?" This question, realized solely with a rise and fall of intonation, is considered biased because the doctor anticipates that the patient will answer affirmatively based on the previous exchange. Jazmín responds according to the doctor's bias not only by nodding but also by repeating the word *normales*. Example 15 illustrates another way in which the doctor uses a biased question as a confirmation strategy:

15) Biased questions

Dr. Ortiz: *¿Ha tomado medicina para esto?*
               Have you taken medication for this? [first question]
Maribel (#10): *No.*
               No.
Dr. Ortiz: *¿No le han dado nada?*
               They haven't given you anything? [second question]
Maribel: *Nuh-uh.*
               Nuh-uh.

The doctor carefully achieves confirmation without repeating the same question. The patient could have interpreted an explicit repetition of the doctor's question as rude and as if the doctor were questioning her judgment or did not believe her. Negative polarity is a subtle way to confirm the response, which helps the doctor maintain a good relationship with the patient.

Example 15 illustrates an additional grammatical resource the doctor uses to displace responsibility from patients, which involves the roles of social actors in the discourse. In the first question, the patient is the subject of that question; she has an active role and is the agent or actor of what is being questioned (taking medicine). However, in his second question, the follow-up/confirmation question ("*¿No le han dado nada?*" "They haven't given you anything?"), he enacts a switch in social roles. In this version, other medical professionals the patient sees replace her as the agent/actor. That is, the question holds the other medical professionals and not the patient responsible for whether the patient takes medication.

At the grammatical level in the second question, the pronoun *ellos* "them" (medical professionals) is the subject, the medication is the direct object, and the patient is the indirect object. Van Leeuwen (2008) describes this strategy as "activation" and "passivation"; in this case, the doctor activates the role of the medical professionals and passivizes that of the patient. By displacing responsibility from the patient and to the other medical professionals, the doctor is signaling that he aligns with the patient and not with the other medical professionals. This alignment is an effort to strengthen his interpersonal relationship with the patient and her trust in him.

Within medical interview genres, biased questions are useful grammatical resources. The doctor needs to collect accurate information from the patient to make appropriate decisions regarding their health care. For these reasons, he needs not only to pose new questions but also to confirm the information. By using negative polarity, the doctor seeks confirmation following the cultural norms of patients and without compromising their doctor–patient relationship.

When confirming information that may be taboo (such as drug use and psychiatric disorders), the doctor commonly uses biased questions. This is not surprising given that, in the genre of psychiatric interviews, discussing sensitive topics pertaining to psychiatric and psychological disorders is commonplace. For example, in the interviews analyzed here, patients and the doctor discussed excessive consumption of drugs and alcohol, medication, food disorders, depression, anxiety, and trauma. These topics are taboo among rural Mexicans, just as they are for many cultures.

Another example of negative polarity concerns eating disorders:

16) Biased questions
Dr. Ortiz: *¿Vomita después de comer?*
             Do you vomit after eating?
Gloria: No.
Dr. Ortiz: *¿Ni usa laxantes ni . . . ?*
             Not even laxatives or . . . ?
Gloria: *Nada, nada.*
             Nothing, nothing.

The doctor could have asked Gloria (female, thirties, #4), "Do you use laxatives?"—and this would have been a more logical rejoinder, as vomiting after eating and using laxatives are different—but instead decides to use negative polarity, and the effect is a more delicate form of raising this topic. By signaling his assumption that the patient will say no, the doctor is also indexing his alignment with her.

The doctor also uses biased interrogatives to avoid excluding patients' potential answers, as shown in example 17, which, as described above, also contains modality:

17) Biased questions

Dr. Ortiz: *¿Cuánto tenía? ¿No le dijo?*
What was your level? Did he not tell you?

Norma: *Me dijo que, se me hace que cien de setentaiuno. Pero me dijo, a la mejor en el futuro puede ser más.*
He told me, I think, 100 over 71. But he told me, maybe in the future it could be more.

The function of the doctor's biased interrogative is to avoid contradicting Norma (female, mid-forties, #12) since the doctor contemplates the possibility that the patient does not know this information. Therefore, by formulating the question using negative polarity, the doctor is creating a safe space for Norma in case she has to say that she does not know. In this case, he is "including" this option and therefore creating inclusivity (as opposed to excluding the option and possibly insulting the patient).

Regarding the social actors involved in the questions, in the first question, *¿Cuánto tenía?* "What did you have?" the patient is the subject and agent. However, in the following question, *¿No le dijo?* "He didn't tell you?" the patient's general practitioner is the subject. The introduction of this new social actor, the agent who is now held responsible for the patient's information, is signaled with the Spanish indirect pronoun "*le.*" As seen in example 15, the doctor activates the role of another medical professional and passivizes the role of the patient to displace responsibility from the patient, avoid putting her on the spot, and align with her.

The doctor uses biased interrogatives for inclusivity to seek information from patients such as weight, height, and physical activity without putting the patient, Carlos (male, mid-sixties, #23) on the spot:

18) Biased questions

Dr. Ortiz: *¿No sabe cuánto pesa?*
You don't know how much you weigh?

Carlos: *No. No. Ah, cuánto peso. Ahorita me pesé aquí. Se me hace que pesé 254 libras.*
No. No. Oh, how much I weigh. I just weighed myself here. I think that I weighed at 254 pounds.

Similarly to the previous example, the doctor creates a safe space in case the patient does not know how much he weighs.

These examples demonstrate how the doctor uses biased interrogatives to create a more inclusive environment regarding patients' potential answers. Consequently, he is protecting patients' self-image (i.e., he is allowing them to save face) by displacing responsibility from them about their health information and other behaviors.

Conclusions

The goal of this chapter has been to illustrate how meaning is realized in a psychiatric interview and to reveal discourse strategies that the doctor uses and how both doctor and patients build a transcultural interpersonal relationship through communication. Findings indicate, for example, that patients used *como* for "semantic loosening" of the information they offered the doctor to explain their symptoms and to draw on comparisons with other similar feelings (Mihatsch 2009). The fuzziness that modality creates makes it easier to cautiously offer medical information to the doctor without being held entirely responsible for that information. The use of these modality devices in medically oriented sections of the interview may indicate how difficult it is to discuss health issues. Patients may also be displaying deference to the doctor based on his medical expertise and profession (Eggins 2004). Indeed, in this medical context, modality is a power mitigation strategy whereby patients index their nonexpert roles in health care compared with the doctor's expert role.

Dr. Ortiz's modality resources aid the interaction in multiple ways. For instance, he uses tag questions as a confirmation strategy while saving face or expressing probability in order to displace responsibility from patients. Bushes in his questions invite patients to make guesses or resort to comparisons. Because he does not want to express that he's unsure about a statement, he avoids using explicit modality devices such as *creo que* "I believe that." Rather, his subtle use makes the patient an active part of the interview process. This is particularly evident when he uses tags as part of confirming answers. By using verbal modality, the doctor works toward creating a less-threatening environment for the patients where communication is more relaxed. He uses it to mitigate the wide power gap between himself and his patients, and thus verbal modality strengthens his interpersonal relationship with patients.

One of the grammatical resources the doctor relies on is constructing biased questions to confirm patient information politely and normalize/

include patients' answers (as opposed to marginalizing them). By making these discourse choices, some of which are face-saving strategies, the doctor builds trust (*confianza*) with his patients and shows respect (*respeto*) (Cordella 2007). Embracing his patients' cultural values, including *confianza* and *respeto,* builds solidarity with them. Such measures are particular vital in psychiatric interviews, since they involve sensitive information, including patients' clinical histories, sociodevelopmental histories, psychiatric symptoms, and substance and alcohol use. For patients to feel comfortable sharing this information with a person they are meeting for the first time, it is crucial that they feel linguistically, culturally, and socially understood. The doctor is successful in forming an effective interpersonal relationship with patients not only because of his transcultural knowledge but also because he uses this knowledge at crucial moments during the interview, as revealed in the discourse.

This chapter illustrates how Dr. Ortiz and his patients employ modality devices and reflect cultural expectations and how the doctor establishes trust and rapport (Allison and Hardin 2020), the foundation of an effective doctor–patient communication. For Latino/a patients, as the literature on Latino health has reported, *respecto* is a crucial cultural construct in working toward good rapport and building trust. This chapter's analysis of politeness strategies gives us contextualized examples of how *respeto* can take place. Strong interpersonal relationships between doctors and patients are associated with patient satisfaction, adherence to treatment, and the course of the illness (Eggly 2002). The evidence suggests that sharing an ethnic background and language and demonstrating transcultural competence is immensely powerful, but there are insights any medical practitioner or interpreter can use here.

Insights for Medical Practitioners and Interpreters

- Politeness and *respeto* go much deeper than knowing when to use the polite versus informal second-person pronouns (*usted/tú*). This chapter offered numerous examples of how Dr. Ortiz uses verbal modality in his questions, a key politeness strategy, to displace responsibility from patients, to pose questions sensitively, and to confirm information. By displacing responsibility from patients and through his sensitivity, the doctor took steps toward gaining their trust, which is vital in a psychiatric interview. Another effect of his use of verbal modality is signaling to patients that using modality is appropriate in the medical context. He leads the way in posing questions carefully and allowing patients to give estimates of their answers should they feel unsure of their responses.

This is an example of how a doctor can use their powerful position to empower patients.

- This chapter also illustrated the reasons for patients' use of verbal modality. Patients use these modality resources recurrently when discussing their symptoms and conditions in order to show deference to the power and expert role of the doctor. The fuzziness that modality creates may make it easier for patients to cautiously offer these details without being held entirely responsible for the information. When a practitioner notices that a patient is using verbal modality, it does not necessarily mean that the patient is unsure of their answer, because modality is a way to express politeness. Awareness of the context of the interaction and actively noticing how people use language gives practitioners more insights into patients' intentions.

- Medical interactions are complex, and how they unfold depends on unpredictable social factors, which vary by context. Given that no two medical interactions are the same, explicit exposure to how these interactions unfold at the language level serves as an exercise in language awareness. This awareness serves as training so that practitioners can make the most of their language choices when pressed for time and/or in high-stakes situations.

CHAPTER 7

Conclusions

Spanish and Transcultural Discourse in Health, Teaching, and Research

THIS BOOK HAS DETAILED ways to address a critical problem in health care today by illustrating how to promote transcultural competence in medical interactions. Latino/a patients in the US face disproportionate risk of health issues including diabetes, AIDS/HIV, cervical cancer, and pesticide poisoning; mistrust in the health care system and language and cultural barriers aggravate their disadvantage (López-Cevallos et al. 2014). Spanish speakers have reported on specific ways to help repair the broken trust with communities such as theirs, recommending that practitioners take time to greet patients, make small talk, and generally aim to connect with them at a human level before the professional level (Magaña 2020). This human-level connection aligns with the cultural constructs of *simpatía, personalismo,* and *respeto* (Cordella 2004; Juckett 2013). When providers break cultural norms, it hinders communication with Latino patients.

Among Dr. Ortiz's patients, Miguel (male, mid-forties, #7), articulates similar concerns. In his interview he says that he has been a farmworker since toddlerhood. The long years of work have caused him serious back pain, and he suffers from depression. But he tells Dr. Ortiz that he has generally avoided medical attention because of language and cultural barriers and the significant limitations of interpreters.

Consultation with Miguel

Miguel: *Eso es el problema que a mí no me gusta. No hay como hablar el idioma de nosotros para decir todos los pecados, dijo el cura. No hay como platicar de persona a persona; no que te estén traduciendo. Y por eso no me gusta atenderme. Ya me enfadé.*

That is the problem that I do not like. There is nothing like speaking in our language to say all of our sins, said the priest. There is nothing like talking from person to person; none of this translating. And that's why I do not like to get seen. I'm tired of this.

Dr. Ortiz has not asked Miguel his feelings about interpreters; clearly, he feels empowered to discuss the impossible situation of using an interpreter in psychiatric care. His quotation of a priest is probably from one he himself knows; thus, he is comparing his interview with Dr. Ortiz to the religious sacrament of confession, a culturally meaningful comparison. Voicing problems in psychiatric interviews is key to proper follow-up care. As this book has demonstrated, transcultural and sociolinguistic knowledge fosters an environment within psychiatric interviews that disposes patients to feel comfortable speaking about their problems.

Carlos (mid-sixties, #23) also articulates the importance of a common language: "*Qué bueno que habla español mero como yo*" (How great that you speak Spanish just like me). As Carlos acknowledges, this is not the norm. His sentiments are reinforced by other Spanish speakers in the US who have called for more Spanish-speaking providers as a way to improve communication issues and build *confianza* in the health care system (Hernández et al. 2011; Magaña 2020). Researchers and health care providers have also offered strong arguments indicating that language-concordant consultations are optimal for patient-centered health care (Fernandez et al. 2011; G. Flores 2006; Ortega 2018).

Sharing patients' language creates opportunities to connect with them. Learning to connect better with Latino communities in the US is crucial for successful interactions and follow-up care (Hansen and Cabassa 2012; Interian et al. 2011). Yet, language is not enough: practitioners must recognize their patients' socialization and histories. For instance, Latino/as may face different layers of discrimination given their minority status, political history, race, socioeconomic status, and level of education. This marginalization may make Latino/a patients feel misunderstood and, in some ways, out of place. Ricardo (male, late forties #21), who has a strong work ethic but is unemployed, has separated from his wife, and deals with alcoholism, articulated this "out of place" feeling. Months before the interview, he developed health issues (he has high blood pressure and diabetes) and was rushed to the hospital during the workday. He describes his resulting feelings to Dr. Ortiz:

Consultation with Ricardo

Ricardo: *Me da desesperación. Me da, pues que, no hallo mi lugar pues.*
          I feel despair. I feel, well, that I can't find my place.

Dr. Ortiz: *¿No halla su lugar?*
          You can't find your place?

Ricardo: [Shakes head].

Such feelings articulate how his situation exacerbates the challenges to his well-being.

Doctors need to carefully handle the connection between themselves and their patients and the negotiation between friendliness and professionalism in psychiatric interviews because patients are vulnerable and may need friendliness. Even differences between a patient's and a doctor's socioeconomic backgrounds alone can pose a barrier in communication and in forming a connection, yet, Dr. Ortiz is largely able to bridge this divide (Bloom-Pojar 2018; Cordella 2004). Nonetheless, medical Spanish education should include training in cross-cultural communication among individuals of different socioeconomic backgrounds, recruitment should seek doctors from lower socioeconomic backgrounds, and health care institutions should treat such backgrounds as a strength. Such training would include language proficiency that spans registers based on their appropriateness in the local community (Colombi and Magaña 2013). Practitioners should have the tools to acknowledge patient's language variety and use transcultural knowledge for meaningful medical interactions. In medical discourse, transcultural competence in the patient's culture and language variety becomes indispensable for practitioners and interpreters since transcultural knowledge plays a crucial role in effective communication between doctors and patients. Transcultural knowledge can have wider benefits beyond the targeted group. For instance, a practitioner who learns to establish *confianza* and *respeto* with her Latino patients may also be a better practitioner for non-Hispanic white (and probably other) patients as well, especially older ones.

Few studies have given deliberate accounts of transcultural communication for local communities of Spanish in the US. We know that this transcultural communication is an advanced capacity that entails grammatical, discursive, strategic, sociolinguistic, and transcultural competence, which can vary across Spanish speakers in the US. By sociolinguistic competence I mean that the practitioner should be able to understand the issues that many Latino/a immigrants in the US face with respect to language, power, society, social class, gender, and education. This advanced proficiency must enable the speaker to participate in their surrounding communities; therefore, ethnolinguistic knowledge of the communities they serve is crucial. The specific linguistic community will vary according to where providers practice, given the diversity among Latino/as. It is essential that practitioners learn informal registers as well as formal registers, given the need to establish communication with local communities.

Medical Spanish courses tend to emphasize vocabulary and some cultural points but tend to take decontextualized approaches (Hardin 2012). Sociolinguistics and transcultural communication could layer and intersect with this instruction by promoting communication skills that help learners accommodate the language to local communities' register and culture in more intentional ways. For example, an advanced second-language learner in a medical Spanish course should be encouraged to learn the cultural elements of the health care approaches of Latino/as in their community (remedies, beliefs, practices, etc.) as well as the terms their patients commonly use. This approach could prepare students and practitioners to use an informal register without any prescriptive attitudes, employing, for example, "sayings" and regional terminology, and expressing cultural knowledge without judgment. As Dr. Ortiz's example suggests, doctors can use this sociolinguistic and transcultural knowledge to form solidarity with these communities and to play an active role in their health care betterment; such knowledge is likely generalizable to a range of disadvantaged, linguistic-minority communities (including speakers of a nonstandard English-language dialect).

As we saw in chapter 5, on register analysis, building interpersonal skills is vital in this effort and requires practitioners to have an awareness of patients' varieties, especially when they use a local or a nonstandard variety. Gaining advanced knowledge of patients' language variety is in line with gaining patient-centered communication skills (Ortega et al. 2020). In general, clinical skills emphasize patient-centered communication, not technical language knowledge, as the principal goal for medical students to practice medicine safely and effectively (Ortega and Prada 2020). This is one reason why medical Spanish courses are beginning to gain attention in medical education (Ortega et al. 2020). Strategies to enhance patient-centered communication skills in medical education are seen as a long-term learning experience that should be adapted according to the communities being served. Ortega and Prada (2020, 253) propose the following strategies for medical language education:

1. using supplemental resources that reflect local linguistic practices (adopting books or glossaries that incorporate such language or creating such resource),

2. partnering with students who have lived experience using local linguistic practices to serve as TAs or course consultants,

3. collaborating with community members as educators (community health workers, advocates, patients, interpreters),

4. implementing service-learning opportunities for students to gain insight into the language use in the local community,

5. integrating course activities that foment local language use (e.g., using ethnolinguistic material, assigning ethnographic observations).

The next section summarizes some of the discourse strategies that Dr. Ortiz uses effectively with patients. A number of these examples are also instances of transcultural communication.

Transcultural Discourse Strategies

In this book's chapters, I have offered a description of the language choices that enable Dr. Ortiz and his patients to communicate within a transcultural context. Using systemic functional linguistics (SFL) theory, the study has explored the linguistic choices available to the doctor in his capacity of creating a transcultural environment for the patient, which is crucial for effective communication in an unfamiliar setting. Some of the strategies he uses are allowing patients to hold the floor, interrupting gently, displaying solidarity (by code-switching, using colloquial terms, offering personal advice, and making personal exchanges), and demonstrating sociolinguistic awareness. The doctor's language choices demonstrate that he is aligning himself with his patients. Within the context of mental health, these strategies are particularly critical given the health disparities that Latino/as face.

Because the doctor and patients are meeting for the first time during the interview, the doctor needs to have an intentional communication approach to get his patients to speak openly about their health concerns. Transcultural communication thus plays an essential role since patients are more willing to discuss their health issues openly in a trustworthy environment. Dr. Ortiz needs to establish *confianza* as quickly as possible. Patients tend to prefer health care providers who are friendly and who explain treatment and diagnoses in ways they understand over those with more impressive credentials;

and language, cultural barriers, and racism may mean that Spanish-speaking Latino patients have greater difficulty than others finding such practitioners (Brenneisen-Goode 2008).

All patients are vulnerable in health care regardless of their immigration status, language, and culture, but Dr. Ortiz's patients are particularly disempowered. Research using discourse analysis has examined this disempowerment (Wodak 1996), including providers' deliberate use of language to create a social distance from their patients (Ainsworth-Vaughn 1998). For instance, some practitioners phrase their communication with patients in the third person instead of the second person (descriptively instead of directly) if other medical personnel is present, one of the most distant styles of communicating with patients. When they fail to greet their patients, this is particularly alienating (Wodak 1996). Such distance objectifies patients and denies them a symmetrical relationship (Wodak 1996). Dr. Ortiz works toward mitigating social distance in a range of ways. As we have seen throughout this book, he uses small talk, personal exchanges, personalization through the use of patients' name and information (e.g., place of birth), humor, and personal advice to establish a more interpersonal relationship with the patient and, as a result, help them feel more comfortable during his interactions with them.

Dr. Ortiz deviates from the exact structure of the questions in his interviews to give them a more conversational feel. These deviations make the interview feel more spontaneous and casual. It also de-emphasizes his control of the interview and his role as expert. One way in which he realizes this spontaneity is by tailoring the questions to each individual. For example, when asking them for their date of birth, he addresses them using their first names, giving the question a more personalized feel.

Even though the doctor and patients are not likely to have a continuing relationship, Dr. Ortiz demonstrates that he is invested in their doctor–patient relationship. He tries to build an interpersonal relationship as if it will last beyond the interview by engaging in personal exchanges, offering patients personal advice, and listening attentively to their stories. When patients have difficulties talking about their childhood experiences, he asks key questions that trigger their stories. With more talkative patients, he gives verbal and nonverbal cues to signal that he is listening. Instances of Dr. Ortiz interrupting a patient are rare. In the cases where he does have to interrupt a patient, he is gentle and strategic in doing so to show *respeto* in order to avoid disrupting or breaking the *confianza* he has built with patients up until that point.

Dr. Ortiz demonstrates "language acceptance" (Martínez 2011) of the patients' varieties. These varieties do not have social prestige and are often stigmatized. However, the doctor demonstrates acceptance of the patients' varieties because he has sociolinguistic awareness of the different varieties spoken in the US and especially those from rural Mexico. His respectful use of colloquialisms and translanguaging practices even when these characteristics may not form part of his own variety reflect this awareness. His demonstration of interest in the patients' varieties by negotiating local terminology and employing these builds *confianza*.

A major factor that makes transcultural knowledge effective in health care settings is that it normalizes people's health perspectives/beliefs. Normalization is a specific technique useful for eliciting sensitive information, which psychiatric interviews require (Carlat 2012). When using Spanish in the US, transcultural knowledge is a necessary precursor to normalization techniques. Demonstrating transcultural knowledge makes people feel seen, heard, and understood. It makes the setting inclusive for the patient. Dr. Ortiz normalizes people's experiences when he demonstrates knowledge of difficult childhoods in rural Mexico (chapter 2) or when he asks questions strategically, as we saw in chapter 6, on politeness, to establish inclusivity and to avoid marginalizing the patients' answers. In mental health care, it is crucial to normalize a topic no matter how out of the ordinary it may be, as seen in the following example with Ramón (male, mid-thirties, #13):

Consultation with Ramón

Dr. Ortiz:	*¿Miras al diablo?*
	You see the devil?
Ramón:	*En veces.*
	Sometimes.
Dr. Ortiz:	*¿Cómo lo ves?*
	How do you see it?
Ramón:	*Una imagen mala.*
	A bad image.
Dr. Ortiz:	*Y, ¿es como qué? ¿Como humano, animal?*
	And, what is it like? Like a human, like an animal?
Ramón:	*Animal.*
	Animal.

Dr. Ortiz maintains a casual tone throughout, and by offering choices ("human" and "animal") demonstrates familiarity with the different forms the devil may take; he normalizes the situation. Thus, he demonstrates transcultural knowledge of the devil in Ramón's religious community (Colombi and

Magaña 2013). This element of the discourse may make Ramón feel more comfortable talking about these experiences, and the doctor's implication that he expects that it may be either human or animal normalizes this understanding.

Dr. Ortiz's ability to treat visions of the devil—which are both strange in his cultural milieu as an educated, upper-middle-class man and a potential signal of severe psychological illness—as normal suggests his vast skill in using discourse strategies to make his patients comfortable and willing to be open. It is equally impressive that he uses a wide range of techniques, ranging from (co-)construction of stories to small talk to personal exchanges to colloquialisms to negative polarity, to make his psychiatric interviews clinically successful.

Medical students who will care for Spanish-speaking and other linguistic-minority patients, as well as health care providers already serving such populations, can extrapolate pedagogical implications from studying his techniques laid out here. Instructors, including medical-Spanish-language instructors, can learn from this study as well. The strategies it has described are particularly fruitful because they are based on authentic medical interactions with numerous examples to illustrate the strategies. Instead of telling students how to interact with patients, these data can serve to show learners how a doctor successfully interacts with his patients. These models can serve as a foundation from which learners can draw and on which they can expand to change or create during their own interactions. Besides teaching the discourse strategies discussed, students also need explicit examples of how transcultural communication, sociolinguistic awareness, and negotiating local varieties are realized at the language level.

Synthesizing Latino Cultural Constructs

Throughout these chapters I have discussed the centrality of normative cultural values, namely, *simpatía, personalismo, respeto,* and *confianza.* These values are not independent of each other but instead overlap. For instance, as noted in chapter 3, on small talk, there is a significant overlap between *personalismo* and *simpatía.* This book has sought to offer specific, contextualized examples of these cultural constructs during real-time doctor–patient interactions. To summarize:

1. Dr. Ortiz shows *simpatía* when he demonstrates attentiveness using verbal and nonverbal cues, as we saw toward the beginning of chapter 2, on genre.

2. He demonstrates *personalismo* and *simpatía* when he engages in small talk or acknowledges patients' conversational offerings (everyday topics, asking about family, etc.). Making small talk in a medical interaction is crucial for creating a comfortable environment and establishing an interpersonal interaction. This is particularly important in the psychiatric interview genre, as patients are expected to speak openly about sensitive issues.

3. He also shows *personalismo* by using humor, giving compliments, and aligning with the patient's positions/views (e.g., through gossip, as shown in chapter 3).

4. His *personalismo* is also revealed when he offers personal advice to patients. For instance, he encourages patients to practice their English and gives information on obtaining prescribed eyeglasses as well as citizenship status (chapter 3).

5. Self-disclosure (discussing his own experiences) is another important way he demonstrates *personalismo*. Dr. Ortiz self-discloses numerous times, specifically when he offers patients advice (both medically and socially oriented) and makes small talk about social matters. Self-disclosure is a technique providers can use to create a more symmetrical relationship and lessen the power gap (chapter 3).

6. He shows *respeto* by making subtle interruptions and allowing patients to complete their turn (in this context, interrupting would imply imposing his agenda and gaining power/control over the discourse), as illustrated in chapter 4, on register.

7. Dr. Ortiz also shows *respeto* by using appropriate address terms using the "*usted*" (formal) form with women and middle-aged men and *tú* with younger men (chapter 4).

8. He is respectful about the patient's preferred language use, for example, avoiding taboo terms and replacing these with culturally appropriate terms (chapter 4).

9. He shows *respeto* by posing questions sensitively (e.g., through posing biased questions using negative polarity, as shown in chapter 6). *Personalismo, simpatía,* and *respeto* can serve to develop *confianza* gradually (Añez et al. 2005). In psychiatric interviews, *confianza* is a key cultural construct.

10. The doctor establishes *confianza* by accommodating patients' speech through the use of colloquialisms to create an informal interaction, as we saw in chapter 5.

11. Similarly, he uses translanguaging practices with bilingual patients (chapter 6). Because the doctor was not socialized in a bilingual setting and

had not spent many years in the US at the time of the interview, his code-switches can be viewed as examples of language accommodation.

12. Another way to create trust is by demonstrating command as a professional (Carlat 2012). Dr. Ortiz does this by guiding the patient throughout the interview (chapter 2) and educating the patient at appropriate times, as we have seen through various examples.

These are some of the recurrent ways in which the doctor demonstrates knowledge of these cultural constructs in the interviews, but there are an infinite number of other ways to achieve *respeto* and *confianza*. My aim here is not to categorize Dr. Ortiz's approaches to these cultural concepts as a fixed list but rather to supplement the literature on cultural constructs in Latino health. These constructs are crucial to building interpersonal relationships between health providers and Latino/a patients and, in turn, improving health care for these patients. Being mindful of these cultural constructs discussed from the start of provider–patient interactions is key, given research on the impact of first impressions; as Añez et al. note, "negative first impression[s] can damage the [doctor–patient] alliance and may predict premature dropout from treatment" (2005, 223). Dr. Ortiz succeeds in forming an interpersonal relationship with patients because of his transcultural knowledge and his *decision* to use this knowledge at crucial moments during the interview.

The examples throughout this book have raised awareness about deliberate ways to deploy Latino values to strengthen connections between what the literature proposes and the specific ways in which this is accomplished. Psychiatric interviews have characteristics that set them apart from other types of medical interactions, involving greater vulnerabilities and trust issues than other interactions, as mental health is particularly personal and almost impossible to measure except by self-report. The way Dr. Ortiz achieves this represents one way among numerous other possible ways depending on the interaction's context. Future research could shed light on cultural constructs across different health care contexts.

Pedagogical Implications

SFL has the potential to help us extrapolate concrete teaching implications from the data presented here, and specific language examples can serve as models and meaning-making possibilities. It offers tools that are appropriate for curricular reform to medical Spanish courses. Instructors for such courses should establish key concepts concerning language ideologies and attitudes deliberately: that language varieties and registers have a functional use, and that there shouldn't be a superiority/inferiority distinction between them since they all have both purpose and function, in line with SFL. Students of medical Spanish should gain sociolinguistic awareness concerning language attitudes, stigma, and the history of these registers. Stigma attached to Spanish and Spanish speakers in the US and other places where Spanish is a minority language increase the need for such instruction if they are to obtain the tools that SFL offers them.

Register theory can help students gain awareness of the distinct registers (context of the situations) in which speakers may be participating: the speakers, what they are talking about, and the mode of communication, all of which influence language choices. These registers can range from a written document to an emergency consultation to nutrition to a physical checkup, to name a few. This would help students understand more explicitly different medical registers to expand on their language uses and therefore navigate these with more ease.

This study's findings indicate that medical Spanish's pedagogical implications should be informed by how successful patient–doctor interactions occur (including how miscommunication is repaired). It is crucial to draw knowledge for best patient-centered care practices using control groups, surveys, interviews, and authentic medical interactions. This book reveals that there is value in colloquial knowledge about health in professional contexts where Spanish is spoken. It is essential that language classrooms on medical Spanish also promote local varieties of the language.

Future Directions

The dialogue between health care providers and language researchers and instructors on best practices for Spanish-language interactions with patients in the US is just beginning, and it signals the need for further collaboration to address communications issues. Doctor training programs should make stronger connections between underserved Latino communities and research within linguistics (especially sociolinguistics and discourse analysis) on Spanish varieties in the US to better serve these communities.

There are many more questions to research concerning how linguistic understanding can help us address disparities in mental health care and health care generally of Latino/as in the US, and I hope studies across different interaction types that have implications for serving more underserved communities in health care will influence medical training, much as I hope this one will. Context affects how language is used, meaning that linguistic choices vary across genres and registers and speakers. Additional research should address the distinct genres of medical interactions such as those occurring between Latino/a patients and nutritionists, gynecologists, therapists, pediatricians, oncologists, emergency department practitioners, and routine consultations. It will also be fruitful to learn how speakers communicate their health concerns across illnesses (e.g., HIV/AIDS, COVID-19, diabetes, cancer) and modalities (virtual consultations, interpreted face-to-face consultations, interpreted video consultations, etc.). Research within these genres will give us a more complete picture of the language situation of Latino/as in health care.

Future research might also systematically study how health information is advertised to Latino/as. Are they directly translated from English, or are they culturally embedded? Is the advice on health care targeted to Spanish speakers inclusive of informal or colloquial registers? We can also continue to gain cultural knowledge by studying how local speakers describe their ailments across different contextualized communication (e.g., during medical visits, in health narratives, and in interactions with family members). This knowledge could also shed some light on disparities in health literacy, which, in the US, are defined from the perspective of the dominant culture. While it is crucial for minority groups to have the linguistic tools needed to access mental health care, it is also important for practitioners to be aware of how local groups of speakers conceptualize mental health issues in their language and culture. This can help ameliorate the cultural barriers that language-minority communities face. Practitioner awareness is particularly crucial given the stigma and cultural construct of *vergüenza* (embarrassment) about mental health issues among Latino groups. Based on this understanding, we can work toward models that would guide treatment and self-management and influence medical adherence. If we understand more about how such groups conceptualize their health, we can give doctors more tools to be culturally and linguistically competent providers. This is also a step toward providing more patient-centered care for medically underserved groups. It is my hope that this book inspires many more studies and ultimately better health care across many communities.

This study has several limitations, including its small sample size and its focus on a specific linguistic community. Having a small sample was valuable to this study because it enabled me to conduct a fine-grained analysis and offer numerous examples. Future research might use a larger corpus and statistical analysis to corroborate the findings suggested here. Future research should also include other Spanish-speaking groups because their language use can vary across numerous sociolinguistic contexts, including ethnicity, socioeconomic status, level of education, and gender identity. How do different groups of Spanish speakers compare with each other in terms of cultural constructs and health care communication? Do newly immigrated Spanish speakers face language and cultural barriers systemically? Are there cultural differences that can lead to further understanding the diversity among Spanish speakers, including indigenous groups? What roles do language and gender play in health care communication in light of cultural constructs of gender in Latino/a communities? How do Spanish-speaking cultures impact communication for men versus women? Answers to these questions require studying health care issues affecting Spanish speakers more robustly and systematically to continue strides in improving health care for all.

It is unreasonable to expect even heritage-Spanish-speaking providers to know everything about the sociocultural situations of the Latino/a patients they care for and to have advanced proficiency in all Spanish-language varieties. Dr. Ortiz, who shares his patients' ethnicity and language, employed imperfect strategies, including minimal efforts to deliberately ask patients whether they have questions and using health metaphors that are common in English but that caused misunderstandings with several of his patients. This book's message is not that practitioners must live up, even, to Dr. Ortiz's impressive (though imperfect) standard. Rather, all practitioners should have be open to how people speak and how cultural constructs are linguistically deployed during consultations. Gaining transcultural knowledge and advanced proficiency in Spanish should be seen as an ongoing learning process. What matters is providers' genuine inclination to learn about people and their language and culture and their ability to gain communication skills that enable them to have an interpersonal relationship that is mutually beneficial, such that patients feel comfortable and providers obtain information necessary for future care. Discourse analysis and inviting the reader to reflect on the language of interviews as this book has done are steps toward developing advanced proficiency and gaining awareness of model examples for conducting transcultural interviews with rural Mexicans and perhaps other communities as well. This awareness serves as training in communication that can be useful in high-stakes situations. Because medical institutions are under pressure to serve many people over short periods, and, as a result, consultations can feel rushed, practitioners must make the most of their language choices.

Given that language-minority groups receive inferior health care delivery, it is crucial to continue discussions about best approaches to patient-centered care for minority groups and enhanced training in culturally and linguistically appropriate communication (McGuire et al. 2012). Addressing this complex issue requires collaboration across multiple stakeholders such as the communities affected, health care providers, community advocates, interpreters, language instructors, and language researchers. These discussions should incorporate feedback directly from the communities affected and include speakers across a wide variety of languages with a focus on those that are underrepresented in health care or who come from marginalized communities. An effective approach in addressing issues that communities of color experience in a more holistic way is community-based participatory research (Deeb-Sossa 2019; Wallerstein et al. 2017). The core principles of community-based participatory research emphasize a cooperative approach in which the community and researchers contribute equally and in which there is a balance between research and action; to achieve this, there must be a co-learning process, a building of community capacity, and the empowering of participants (Wallerstein et al. 2017). Indeed, communities affected by health care barriers are the experts on those barriers and on how to overcome them. Therefore, identifying their knowledge and giving them a voice will shed light on the best approaches to advocacy and community interventions (Deeb-Sossa 2019). For example, an academic partnership with a community health organization can help create an infrastructure to involve stakeholders in developing a plan for improving provider and interpreter training based on participants' recommendations. Giving voice to local communities is not only a more humane approach to addressing problems in health care communication; it can also offer insightful solutions if we as researchers and practitioners choose to listen.

APPENDIX I

Summary of Patients' Backgrounds

THE FOLLOWING IS brief information about each patient and his or her health circumstances. All patients emigrated from Mexico unless otherwise noted. To protect their anonymity, all names are pseudonyms.

Josefina is a woman in her late forties. She is a married homemaker. She expresses multiple symptoms of anxiety and depression, including being sad, crying easily, and feeling uneasy and sleepy all day. She acknowledges that she is constantly worried and afraid that something bad is going to happen without a reasonable cause. She also feels a slight pain in her liver and feels that her stomach is going to burst. She worries about her teenage children and gangs her in neighborhood. Her worries are so severe that sometimes she vomits.

Alma is in her mid-sixties. She used to work as a farmworker but is now disabled and unemployed. She is married. In addition to depression, she deals with diabetes and high blood pressure. She has dealt with interpersonal issues with her daughter-in-law, who Alma says mistreats her.

Guadalupe is one of four Mexican American patients. She was raised in the Central Valley. Guadalupe describes having a difficult childhood because of her mother's abandonment of her and her siblings. Her grandmother raised her and was very strict. She has dealt with numerous health issues: a gallbladder procedure, pancreas attacks, memory loss from an accident, diabetes, and kidney cancer. She exercises regularly, has hobbies, and has a good support system through friends and her grown children.

Gloria, mid-thirties, is a married woman. She has worked as a janitor but is unemployed at the time of the interview. Her symptoms point to anxiety and depression. She explains that she has trouble feeling at ease. She says that she is very emotional, cries easily, and has had suicidal thoughts. Her brother's suicide and the fact that some of her family still live in Mexico has caused her a great deal of grief.

Pilar is in her mid-thirties and is on maternity leave. She has a newborn and two other children. Pilar is a field-worker and is married. She describes dealing with postpartum depression after her first child was born, for which she never sought treatment because she didn't understand it. She cries easily and feels great sadness.

Alejandro is a Mexican American man in his mid-thirties born and raised in the Central Valley. He is single and works as a construction worker. He identifies as gay but kept this a secret until he left his parents' home at age nineteen. He deals with symptoms of anxiety and depression (loss of sleep, social isolation, lack of grooming, suicidal thoughts). He describes being raised in a home with alcoholism and physical and emotional abuse.

Miguel is in his mid-forties and lives with his girlfriend. He has worked as a farmworker all his life. He had a difficult childhood because of an abusive father and extreme poverty. His stressors include financial instability and pressure to financially help his parents in Mexico. He describes getting depressed and having suicidal thoughts, which he attributes to "mental weakness."

Roberto, early forties, is a field-worker and lives with his girlfriend. He worries a lot about his parents in Mexico. His mother is ill and depends on his financial support. Like Miguel, he attributes his mental health conditions to "weakness from the brain." He says it is hard for him to find joy in things that he used to enjoy.

Juan is a man in his early forties. He works at a restaurant and is married, but his wife lives in Mexico with their three children. He experiences sadness because of family separation and loneliness. He says he copes by drinking and by engaging in casual sexual encounters and that he used to use illegal drugs.

Maribel is a woman in her mid-forties. She is a widow who used to work in the packaging industry but now receives government disability payments. She says she has dealt with depression since she was ten years old. She has suicidal thoughts. She worries about her son, and his problems stress her out.

Trinidad is a retired woman in her mid-sixties who worked in the fields. She is separated from her husband. She worries constantly about the welfare of their children and often feels frustrated. Her health issues include diabetes, high blood pressure, and depression. She's also worried about memory-loss issues.

Norma is a married woman in her mid-forties. She had a difficult upbringing in rural Mexico, including being sexually abused by her stepfather when she was a child. She works in the fields. She has prediabetes, severe headaches, and sleep issues, and she deals with depression. One of her main stressors is problems with one of her daughters, who is involved in gangs.

Ramón is a Mexican American man in his mid-thirties. He is single, lives with his mother, and is unemployed. His father beat him with a cable wire or with a whip when he was a child. In addition to describing depression and mania, he has high blood pressure and some liver issues. He has never received treatment for a mental health illness, even though his case seems severe. He says he sees and hears voices speaking to him and has heated arguments with people on the street. He has sleep issues and avoids going out because he is scared that people will be mad at him.

José is a man in his mid-fifties. He has a persistent stutter. He had a difficult upbringing. His father was abusive. He is taking multiple medications for pain, balance/dizziness issues, and convulsions. He often trails off during his answers to the doctor's questions.

Jazmín is a married woman in her late twenties. She has dealt with depression since the birth of her child (who at the time of the interview is four years old). She has difficulty getting out of bed, eats compulsively, and experiences headaches.

Teresa is a married woman in her early fifties. She is unemployed and previously worked in a packaging plant. Teresa deals with numerous issues in her family, including her husband's severe diabetes and her sons' addiction to drugs. Her own health issues are diabetes, breast cancer, depression, and anxiety. She believes her family's circumstances have triggered her depression. During the interview Teresa describes a suicide attempt.

Martín is a man in his early fifties. He is divorced and unemployed. He explains that he has been dealing with depression for two years. He began to isolate himself when he lost his job two years ago, and attributes his depression to this, his job loss, and his marital and financial problems. He says that depression causes him to feel a lack of motivation and sadness. He has suicidal thoughts.

María is a woman in her mid-forties. She has worked as a house cleaner, but at the time of the interview she is unemployed. She deals with depression. She believes her son is involved with drugs and gangs, and his problems are her main stressors.

Érica is a woman in her mid-thirties. She lives with her partner but has difficulties with that relationship. She is unemployed and has depression. She was married at a young age but got divorced. She has a seventeen-year-old daughter from that marriage who lives with her father. Érica had an abortion because of pressure from her current boyfriend. She became pregnant again but had a stillbirth. This has caused her great sadness and issues with her partner.

Amalia is a woman in her seventies. Even though she lives with her husband, she explains that they do not have a good relationship and that he mistreats her. They sleep in different rooms and he calls her crazy. She feels that most of her thirteen children, who do not visit or call her, do not value her. Her health issues are diabetes and depression.

Ricardo is a man in his late forties. He is separated from his wife. At the time of the interview he is unemployed. He deals with alcoholism, diabetes, high blood pressure, and depression. He has suicidal thoughts but seeks support from his church and his friends.

Cesar is a Mexican American man in his mid-thirties. He's married and has six children. He was raised on a ranch by strict parents who hardly went out in public and who often restricted his movements. He deals with severe anxiety and panic attacks. He has trouble being in public or at social gatherings and has sleep problems.

Carlos is a divorced man in his mid-sixties. He used to work in the fields but at the time of the interview is unemployed and financially dependent on his four grown children. He deals with anxiety, leg and foot pain, and high blood pressure. He is on medication, and because he is illiterate he uses tally marks to indicate how much medicine to take.

Sample of a Complete Interview

THE INITIAL GREETINGS were not recorded in this interview. Potential identifiers have been replaced with brackets.

Small Talk

Amalia: Es que somos una familia muy grande y todos salieron adelante.

Dr. Ortiz: ¿Y por qué no los quieren?

Amalia: Por eso. Por que somos mexicanos y somos los [inaudible] según.

Dr. Ortiz: ¿Quince hijos y todos le salieron buenos?

Amalia: Si, gracias a Dios. Son nueve mujeres y seis hombres.

Dr. Ortiz: Uno le descompusieron pero se va a componer.

Amalia: Ese me lo descompusieron.

Dr. Ortiz: Se va a componer, va a ver.

Amalia: Lo que pasa es que yo he sufrido muchísimo con mi esposo porque mi esposo es un mexicano muy machista. A mi nunca me ayudó él con nada, oiga. Yo trabajé día y noche para sacar a mis hijos adelante.

[00:00:59]

Dr. Ortiz: ¿De verás?

Amalia: Me iba en la noche, a trabajar. Y en el día duré tiempo, como seis años.

Interview Procedure

Doctor: Mire, primero le voy a hacer como una consulta como la que le da [doctor's name] pero va a haber énfasis en sus problemas psicológicos. Luego le voy a hacer estas preguntas y usted me debe contestar con sí o no nada más. Eso es lo que vamos a grabar en el video. Ya después apagamos la cámara y dependiendo de lo que me haya dicho aquí tenemos que ver algunas de estas secciones.

Amalia: Oh, OK.

[00:00:30]

Demographic Information

Dr. Ortiz: ¿En [year] nació?

Amalia: Sí. Estoy muy viejita.

Dr. Ortiz: Se ve como de cincuenta, como de mi edad.

Amalia: Tengo setentaidós años. [Risas] Bien acabados.

Dr. Ortiz: ¿Qué religión tiene?

Amalia: Soy católica 100 por ciento hasta ahorita.

Dr. Ortiz: Todos los mexicanos no la cuidan, ¿verdad? Todos los demás se hacen cristianos.

[00:01:32]

Amalia: Tenemos ese—desde que abrimos los ojos somos católicos.

Dr. Ortiz: Y aquí la de—¿Y sigue casada?

Amalia: Sí. ¿Sé imagina cincuentaicuatro años de casada?

Dr. Ortiz: Pues sí.

[00:01:59]

Amalia: [Risa] Y con el mismo dice. Ay, pero que golpe. Así es.

History of Present Illness

Dr. Ortiz: ¿Y entonces porque se deprime tanto?

Amalia: Mire, me da mucha depresión por mi marido porque él no me apoya para nada. Para él yo no valgo, yo estoy loca, yo nomás quiero cosas buenas y no es verdad que quiero cosas buenas porque si yo—ahorita ya estamos retirados, ya no puedo trabajar.

[00:02:29] Desde que me salió un tumor tan grande y luego enseguida me dio el stroke, me dio un ataque al corazón, pues ya definitivamente. Y dice, tú nomás quieres puras cosas buenas, yo no puedo dártelas. Le digo, nunca me las has dado. Sí me gusta lo bueno.

No lo niego, pero hasta donde puedo, hasta donde alcanzo. Y es mucho sufrir. Tenemos separados ya de cuarto, de todo. Vivimos juntos pero—pero ya no somos esposos.

[00:03:03] Tenemos 13 años. Entonces yo tengo muchas cosas que a veces—que me paro en la puerta de su cuarto. A veces tengo tanto miedo en mi cuarto que alguien habló, ay escucho algo. Me voy con mi pillow en la mano, le digo, ¿me dejas quedarme contigo? No. [Se encoge de hombros y cruza brazos]. Me regreso y me pongo a llorar mucho porque digo, ¿por qué yo el ando rogando?

[00:03:31] No tengo porqué hacer eso. Y ya me digo, Dios mío, dame fuerzas. Yo no tengo porque rogarle.

Dr. Ortiz: ¿Ninguno de sus hijos vive con ustedes ya?

Amalia: Ahorita ya están dos.

Dr. Ortiz: ¿Dos?

Amalia: Por que perdieron su trabajo también. [Inaudible] con un rancho, se quebró una mano y un pie y pues tuvieron miedo que les fuera a levantar, que eso era un [inaudible] y de todos modos le quitaron el trabajo. Pero este entonces ya pusimos la casa a nombre de él.

[00:04:05] Entonces estamos viviendo nosotros ahí, pero es de él la casa. Se llama Jorge. Y ahorita uno que anda de troquero, que siempre está ahí a veces. Ahorita se sale a trabajar y regresa pero ahí están dos. Estábamos solos completamente pero es una cosa que yo no puedo soportar porque yo me he portado bien toda mi vida, ¿entonces por qué salimos con eso ahora?

[00:04:31] Yo no puedo entender. El es mayor que yo, cinco, casi seis años. Que se mira mejor que yo, quizá sí porque pues él no se preocupa por nada. Yo fui la que—como yo, cuando mis hijas estaban todas en la escuela yo decía, mis hijas tienen que estar diciendo "ey" porque oigo muchas que hasta una palabra fea usan, "oye, güey, ey cómprame una troca." Mis hijas no tienen que hacer eso. En el field trabajaba yo día y noche y ahora que ellas ganan mucho porque la que es detective pues gana más o menos buen dinero.

La otra ahorita es la que anda patrullando, que apenas tiene dos años de policía. Ella trabaja en [city name]. Está ganando ahorita un dineral porque trabaja para dos escuelas y como ahorita hay graduaciones y todo eso, trabaja muchísimo.

[00:05:30] Pero oiga, esa ni siquiera—ni siquiera una llamada me da. Entonces yo diario estoy deprimida, llorando, por todos y a veces digo, no tiene caso. Pero el sentimiento así es.

Dr. Ortiz: Que raro que tantos hijos educados a la mexicana y que no la vean.

Amalia: Esa niña que anda ahorita patrullando en [city name] y este que es troquero, él vino de un año aquí y la muchachita tenía tres años. Los demás tres, cuatro, cinco—todos hicieron su escuela aquí. No a menos de que ella—pues venían grandes—

Dr. Ortiz: Sí, pero la casa era mexicana.

Amalia: Exactamente. Era mexicana y ella sigue siendo mexicana pero ellas ya se casaron con americanos. Entonces, no sé porque se les ha subido a la cabeza todo eso.

[00:06:30]

Dr. Ortiz: Lo que pasa es que así es la gente aquí.

Amalia: Ay no.

Dr. Ortiz: Se van y ya no regresan, y si pueden se van lo más lejos que se pueda de los papás.

Amalia: Yo les digo a todas las mamá que ahorita están con sus hijas, que sufren bastante porque yo—no me tocó eso. Les digo, no se preocupen ustedes tanto por sus hijos en darles todo, él que se va a la universidad ya no regresa a la casa. Así me pasó así. El que se gradúa, se va a la universidad; ya no regresa.

[00:07:02]

Dr. Ortiz: Lo que uno quiere es que vayan para que hagan algo en la vida, ¿no?

Amalia: Como mi hijo el más pequeño. Lo tuve de cuarentaicinco años el más chiquito. Este nomás se graduó, no ha terminado su carrera. El se fue a la Marina. En cuanto se graduó de high school, se fue a la Marina. [Inaudible] y regresó. Estuvo cinco años en la Marina. Regresó pero—y muy bien. El sí está muy bien porque tiene educación aunque no dejó el estudio por irse hasta la escuela, trabaja y estudia.

[00:07:37]

Dr. Ortiz: Sí, la [person's name] les da mucho—

Amalia: Sí, ahorita—creo que tenía una entrevista, me dijo ayer porque el me llama a diario. El que vive allá en [state name], me dice, mañana tengo un appointment para—quiero trabajar para el gobierno federal, me quiero cambiar al federal; si me dan el trabajo ahorita pues lo agarro porque yo ya me cansé de ser, dice, de ser narcótico.

[00:08:07] Ya me enfadé de andar diario—no traemos ni chaleco—

Dr. Ortiz: Sí, no porque andan de incógnito.

Amalia: Exacto. Dice, nada más traemos pistola pero andamos arriesgando mi vida. No. No. No, pero así. Pero como estábamos tan bien entrenados les mirábamos hasta—como que en los ojos les hemos de ver cuando [inaudible], no.

[00:08:36] Y dice, si no me dan trabajo ahorita me voy a dejar—me voy a salir del trabajo por dos años para terminar mi escuela; si acabo, mientras la Marina, me pague puedo estudiar a donde yo quiera. Y eso es un consuelo que tengo porque es el más chiquito y es él que está más estruido y piensa mucho en mi.

[00:09:03] No, cuando estaba en Irak decía, mejor no como para llamarle. A ella [inaudible] nueve meses en Irak y se imagina, yo nomás en ese tiempo no dormía, yo nomas mirando televisión, todos vestidos igual, ¿ya me matarían al mío? No sé, pero gracias a Dios si regresó. Pero digo yo, ¿por qué este?

[00:09:30] ¿Será porque tuvo muchas cosas en la vida? ¿Qué ya miró mucho? No se ha retirado de mi y a veces hasta mis yernos me dicen, ya déjelo, él ya está casado y todo. Yo no lo detengo, yo no le digo, llámame todos los días. El es el que quiere estar sabiendo de mí. Y por eso se parece tanto a mí que dice, ay Dios [inaudible]. Pero sí, sí tengo muchos, mucho sentimiento dentro de mí que hay veces que quisiera—me tomo pastillas, oiga que a veces no sé ni que es lo que me tomo en la noche.

[00:10:08] He estado—

Dr. Ortiz: ¿Para dormir?

Amalia: Sí, para dormir ya sé cual tomo pero hay veces que yo me siento tanto, tanto, tan mal que me digo, bueno, esa no me hizo efecto. Me voy a tomar otra de estas y otras de estas otras. Y las últimas me da mucha ansiedad [agita manos], me levanto, camino, me tiro. No sé que hacer.

[00:10:30] Ay, Dios, no, y es una tensión. Amanezco sin dormir, me paso sentada. Ahorita está una de mis hijas que vive en México. Esa se fue a México y ya casada aquí, se llevó una niña de aquí y se fue a vivir a México y ahorita vino. Está aquí y duerme en otra—en el mismo cuarto que el mío nomás que en otro—así. Y yo sentada en la noche.

[00:11:03]   Y ayer se despierta, ¿amá, que está haciendo? No puedo dormir. Ay, amá, duérmete. No puedo. [Ve Kleenex en su mano y se limpia cara]. Me pongo tan, tanto, tan nerviosa, le digo. Ya me tomé—tómate una pastilla. Ay, mija, ya me he tomado seis ahorita y mira, no me sirven de nada. Y es una cosa que es lo que yo quisiera—estuve tomando mucho—como por unos cuatro años estuve tomando esa pastilla, la Parcel.

[00:11:33]

Dr. Ortiz: ¿La Parcel?

Amalia: Yeah, pero ya el doctor dijo, no, esto ya no.

Dr. Ortiz: ¿Por qué no? Es muy buena.

Amalia: Dice que agarra a uno adicta. Eso fue lo que me dijo el doctor. Dice, no quiero que se me haga adicta a esa pastilla.

Dr. Ortiz: ¿Le servía?

Amalia: Oh, sí. Esa si me servía. [Cruza la pierna]. Pero el dijo que me hacía adicta y que no quería tener una persona y—le digo, sólo Dios.

[00:12:02]

Dr. Ortiz: ¿Cuánto tiempo tiene de no tomarla?

Amalia: Ahorita ya tengo cuatro años porque ya hasta el doctor se murió antes que yo. Estaba un poquito más—será unos cinco o cuatro años más grande que yo, pero él según me cuidaba mucho. Ay, mi señora, la tengo que cuidar porque—mirar bien lo que hace falta. El se murió en un ratito de un ataque al corazón y yo aquí estoy todavía. Ya cuando me dio a mí el ataque al corazón, ya ni estaba él.

Substance Abuse and Past Medical History

Dr. Ortiz: ¿Y para dormir que toma?

Amalia: [Busca en su bolsa] Ay, ahorita estoy tomando una para dormir. De pura causalidad la traigo aquí porque se me terminó y dije, voy a—esta es la que tomo para dormir [entrega frasco a doctor]. Y sí, sí me funciona hasta ahorita. No del todo como yo quisiera porque hay veces que tengo que tomar otras cosas, hasta té o algo pero esa si me está funcionando.

Dr. Ortiz: Pero ya se le acabó.

[00:13:03]

Amalia: Ya se me acabó.

Dr. Ortiz: ¿Tiene refill todavía?

Amalia: Tiene uno, pero voy a decirle—porque aquí trabaja una de mis hijas.

Dr. Ortiz: ¿Ah, si?

Amalia: Sí, se llama [daughter's name], una morenilla que se parece a mí.

Dr. Ortiz: No, es que como no vengo más que a—bueno, vengo dos veces a la semana pero estoy aquí todo el tiempo, no las conozco a todas.

Amalia: Sí, aquí trabaja ella y le voy a decir que le diga a mi doctor que le haga mejor una receta porque si él llama no me las dan tan pronto.

[00:13:31] Y si yo llevo la receta si—

Dr. Ortiz: Claro. ¿Toma alcohol?

Amalia: No.

Dr. Ortiz: ¿Drogas?

Amalia: No, de ninguna. Yo pienso—

Dr. Ortiz: ¿Cuánto mide?

Amalia: Mido 5"4. Era yo alta. Era alta, yo pero ya—

Dr. Ortiz: ¿Cuánto pesa? [25]

Amalia: Peso—ay, ahorita traigo mucho peso de más, 165 libras.

Sociodevelopmental History

Dr. Ortiz: ¿Dónde nació?

Amalia: En Jalisco, México.

Dr. Ortiz: ¿En qué parte de Jalisco?

Amalia: En una ciudad que se llama [city name].

Dr. Ortiz: Yo soy chilango.

Amalia: Ah, que bien. La familia de uno de mis yernos es de México también. Yo fui a México—

Dr. Ortiz: Nada más que apenas tengo tres años aquí, ¿cómo ve?

Amalia: Está bien.

Dr. Ortiz: Ya me vine bien viejo.

Amalia: No, usted no está viejo.

Dr. Ortiz: Cincuentaisiete años acabo de cumplir.

Amalia: Fíjese cincuentaisiete, yo tengo un hijo de cincuentaitrés. ¿Se imagina?

Dr. Ortiz: ¿Oiga y cómo fue su infancia allá en Jalisco?

Amalia: Muy mala.

Dr. Ortiz: ¿Sí?

Amalia: Económicamente, no. Lo que pasa es que mi mamá fue muy descuidada con nosotras. Nos dejó muy pequeñas y fue muy mala la vida por eso yo me casé a los diecisiete años porque según yo me quería—

[00:15:00]

Dr. Ortiz: Salir.

Amalia: Quería que alguien mirara por mí porque mi mamá nos dejó. Yo tenía ocho años. Cuando mi mamá nos dejó había otro más pequeño que yo, de cinco.

Dr. Ortiz: ¿Cuántos eran en total?

Amalia: Éramos seis.

Dr. Ortiz: ¿Seis?

Amalia: Sí, y mi mamá fue muy descuidada. Se volvió a casar después, primero se fue con el hombre, nos dejó solas, teníamos todo. Teníamos todo, teníamos vacas, teníamos todo pero estábamos chiquillas.

[00:15:30]   Y, usted sabe que eso es lo que no—no puedo. Ya perdoné a mi mamá, ¿no?, en mi mente pero [inaudible] estaba muy chiquito, de siete años.

Dr. Ortiz: OK.

Amalia: Y yo desde entonces—ya murió mi madre y me dolió mucho su mente porque ni siquiera fui. Ya estaba yo aquí cuando murió ella, pero con él yo nunca he vuelto a hablar. No quiero hablar de eso, yo lo perdoné en una—en un retiro pero sé que ahí—

[00:16:07]

Dr. Ortiz: Claro, algo se queda.

Amalia: Sí. Sí.

Medical History

Dr. Ortiz: ¿Alguna vez ha estado en consulta con el psiquiatra o psicólogo?

Amalia: No, nada más una vez por eso, porque me mandó mi doctor porque entonces—¿ahorita que serán? Como nueve años, porque mi esposo tenía un amante al lado y yo según me quería ir de la casa y ni me fui.

Small Talk

[00:16:34] Me fui a [city name] con mi hija que ya está casada con un americano.

Dr. Ortiz: ¿Allá vive?

Amalia: Allá vive. Ahorita está haciendo su carrera para doctora y me fui—

Dr. Ortiz: [Inaudible]

Amalia: No, ella vive en [city name].

Dr. Ortiz: ¿Sí? ¿Pero en que escuela?

Amalia: Ella está para—ahorita está trabajando—parece que está yendo a [name of a college].

Dr. Ortiz: ¿No hay otra escuela? Es la única escuela de medicina.

[00:17:01]

Amalia: Va a empezar ella apenas el semestre que empieza porque está—y ahorita hizo hasta un—habían agarrado otra casa y ella dijo—

Dr. Ortiz: Yo soy maestro ahí en la escuela de medicina.

Amalia: Ah, fíjese que bien. Mi hija se llama [person's name].

Dr. Ortiz: Sí, voy a fijarme.

Amalia: Si es que va ahí porque dice, no me agarra tan lejos. Estaba ella tratando de venirse a Visalia porque es más barato.

[00:17:37]

Dr. Ortiz: Pero aquí no hay escuela de medicina.

Amalia: No, pero ella iba a venir a agarrar su—porque ella trabaja y ella estudia al mismo tiempo porque les están dando—o sea les dan la oportunidad. Ella es muy güerita, güerita también. Pero ella dice, yo no sé amá, no sé, la verdad; ahorita estoy entre la espada y la pared porque me va a costar mucho dinero este estudio y allá en Visalia que se iba a venir a Bakersfield, más bien. Pero no le gustó en Bakersfield. Ya fue a mirar el colegio, a la escuela de Bakersfield, y dice, no me gustó allá. Preferiría agarrar mis primeras clases en Visalia y luego ya cambiarme para acá a [inaudible], se me haría más—pero cómo se va a cambiar ella para acá, ¿y sus niños?

[00:18:30] El es maestro. No. No me sé el nombre de su—pero él es maestro de escuela también. El trabaja ahí mismo en [city name]. Y yo le digo, pues no puedes dejar a los niños allá, y tu esposo y tú acá.

Dr. Ortiz: No.

Amalia: ¿Cómo? No, pues que con tiempo tenemos que mirar para que marche—pues se quieren ir para allá.

Dr. Ortiz: Que pida su cambio.

Amalia: Que pida su cambio, le digo. Eso ahorita es imposible, como está el tiempo ahorita que hasta quieren descansar tantísimos maestros. Entonces ella dice, pues entonces no me va a quedar otra más que—dice, sí me aceptaron ya. Ya me llegaron mis papeles que si me aceptaron. Pero es mucho el dinero que tengo que pagar. Y habían comprado una casa, bueno ya—dice, ya también está el cheque en la mano, de real state que hicimos el trato, ¿y sabe qué? No.

[00:19:30] Le digo, porque me empezó a poner cosas de más y yo me traté viendo, viendo esos papeles minuciosamente, dijo y ahí hay cuentas que no habíamos hablado. Entonces, le dije, ¿sabe qué? Déjese esto. Y ya fue donde ya no hubo trato. Dice, y luego yo mejor me puse a pensar; le dije a mi esposo, ¿sabes que? Si compramos esta casa, olvídate de mi estudio. Yo no voy a poder estudiar. No pues, sabes qué, mejor—

[00:20:00]

Dr. Ortiz: ¿En qué parte de [city name] vive?

Amalia: Vive en [region name].

Dr. Ortiz: Ah, pues ahí vivo yo, en [region name].

Amalia: Ella vive. La calle por donde ella vive se llama [person's name], sí, parece que [person's name].

Dr. Ortiz: Nosotros vivimos en un complejo nuevo que hicieron, tiene como 3 años, que se llama [person's name].

Amalia: Ah, no.

Dr. Ortiz: Pero está en [region name].

[00:20:29]

Amalia: Pues yo conozco poquito porque nomás duré tres semanas con ella. Sí voy y la visito pero—porque aunque inclusive ahorita no está del todo bien su operado de—

Dr. Ortiz: ¿De un hombro?

Amalia: De un hombro, pues ya le operaron los dos. Sí.

Dr. Ortiz: A mí también ya me operaron los dos hombros.

Amalia: Y esta que vive en [city name] le operaron ya las dos rodillas.

Dr. Ortiz: Rodillas.

Amalia: Y le tienen que remplazar una parte. Esa fue por una caída por andar siguiendo a un guy. Dice, él brinco y yo dije, yo brinco también.

[00:21:03]   Y pues yo brinqué, pero caí y me lastimé. Dice, ya el fulano que iba siguiendo, dijo, se agarró riéndose y ya me puso de nuevo las esposas y [inaudible] se cayó.

Dr. Ortiz: ¿A la policía le tienen que cambiar una rodilla?

Amalia: Sí.

Dr. Ortiz: ¿Una prótesis?

Amalia: Sí, tienen que cambiarle una.

Dr. Ortiz: Quedan muy bien eh.

Amalia: Y ella es—está pesadita, está bien—sí, no gorda pero sí está grande y bien fuerte. Y esta, ahorita ella anda aliviada de su rodilla.

[00:21:32]   Inclusive mañana dijeron que se iban a ir a Disneylandia, pero yo no sé les digo, ya no sirven ustedes. Yo que tengo tanto año, mírenme, lo único que tengo es, pues, hay cosillas así pero—

Medical History

Dr. Ortiz: ¿Alergias tiene usted, algo?

Amalia: No.

Dr. Ortiz: ¿Fuma?

Amalia: No.

Dr. Ortiz: ¿Café?

Amalia: No. Ah, café si tomo.

Dr. Ortiz: ¿Cuántos?

Amalia: Nomás en la mañana.

Dr. Ortiz: ¿Uno?

[00:22:00]

Amalia: Sí, un cafecito y descafeinado.

Dr. Ortiz: Ah, entonces no toma café.

Amalia: No, café con cafeína no.

Dr. Ortiz: Puras mentiras.

Amalia: No, con cafeína no. Descafeinado.

Dr. Ortiz: ¿Toma otras medicinas aparte de esas?

Amalia: Sí, tomo muchas pero no me las traje. Soy diabética también. Aparte de esta tomo como otras ocho medicinas. Tomo mucha medicina.

Dr. Ortiz: Pues está muy bien para ser diabética.

[00:22:29]

Amalia: Sí, soy diabética, pues gracias a Dios—no, yo siento que ya no. Ahorita ya ni ando mal. Tengo que componerme o ya me voy definitivamente. Yo estoy ya bien decidida y yo le digo a Dios todos los días, yo estoy lista. Yo espero ya—

Sociodevelopmental History

Dr. Ortiz: ¿Nietos, bisnietos?

Amalia: Nietos tengo treintaiún y bisnietos tengo tres.

Dr. Ortiz: ¿Tataranietos?

Amalia: No, están chiquitos los bisnietos.

Dr. Ortiz: ¿Sí?

[00:23:04]

Amalia: Están chiquitos pero—

Dr. Ortiz: Treintaiún nietos.

Amalia: Treintaiún nietos y eso es que este muchachito, este que vive allá en Arizona, no tiene hijos. Ya tienen cinco años de casados. Se casó a los veintiún años. Y luego estos otros dos que están en la casa están solteros, no tienen hijos tampoco. Otra, la que trabaja en Fresno no tiene hijos tampoco, si no ya tuviera cincuenta yo creo.

[00:23:28]   Y luego me dicen—mucha gente me dice, ay señora, ¿por qué tiene tanto hijo? ¿No había televisión? Le digo, gracias a Dios, si hubiera habido televisión, tantísimas cosas que se ven ahí; hubiera tenido cincuenta, cincuenta hijos.

Screening of Psychiatric Disorders

Dr. Ortiz: Le voy a leer unas preguntas.

Amalia: A ver, dígame.

Dr. Ortiz: Y me contesta sí o no. ¿Ha estado constantemente deprimida o sin ánimos la mayor parte del tiempo las últimas dos semanas?

Amalia: Oh, sí.

Dr. Ortiz: ¿En las últimas dos semanas le ha bajado mucho el interés de las cosas o no disfruta las cosas que antes disfrutaba?

[00:24:02]

Amalia: No, no disfruto nada porque no tengo ocasión—no tengo ni— [mira a los pies].

Dr. Ortiz: ¿Se ha sentido triste, sin ánimos o deprimida la mayor parte del tiempo los últimos dos años?

Amalia: Sí, es cuando me ha dado más duro.

Dr. Ortiz: ¿En el mes pasado se sintió que estaría mejor muerta o deseó estar muerta?

Amalia: Pues hay veces que si deseo pero luego me pongo a pensar, pero—pues como que sí porque pienso que en el otro mundo voy a encontrar unas cosas mejores. Eso pienso yo.

[00:24:35]

Dr. Ortiz: ¿Alguna vez en su vida ha tenido—ha estado así como muy high, con mucha energía, que se haya metido en problemas legales o con la gente?

Amalia: No.

Dr. Ortiz: ¿Peleonera?

Amalia: No. No. No. Soy bien tonta.

Dr. Ortiz: ¿Ha tenido ataques o crisis que de pronto se siente ansiosa, asustada o inquieta en situaciones que otra gente no se sentiría así?

Amalia: Yo pienso que sí y es cuando tomo más pastillas. Sí me siento mal.

[00:25:03]

Dr. Ortiz: OK. ¿Se siente inquieta o ansiosa en lugares en las que no puede salir fácil o en las que hay mucha gente o—

Amalia: No.

Dr. Ortiz: ¿En el mes pasado ha tenido pensamientos o imágenes desagradables, inadecuadas o dolorosas?

Amalia: No.

Dr. Ortiz: ¿En el mes pasado ha hecho algo repetidamente sin poder dejar de hacerlo como lavarse las manos y volvérselas a lavar y otra vez?

[00:25:34]

Amalia: Bueno, sí porque decían que sí no se lavaba las manos a cada ratito me daba la—

Dr. Ortiz: ¿La influenza?

Amalia: La influenza, sí. Sí.

Dr. Ortiz: ¿Alguna otra cosa?

Amalia: No.

Dr. Ortiz: Así que repita muchas veces.

Amalia: Lo que—hay veces que lo que me da mucho es por bañarme. Tomo el shower porque siento que me relajo. Inclusive si ando así como temblorosa, siento que me da—me ayuda.

[00:26:00]

Dr. Ortiz: No toma, no drogas, su edad y su peso ya los tengo. ¿Ha tenido periodos en los últimos tres meses de comer mucho, comer de más?

Amalia: Ay, como que sí. No sé por qué. Sí. Sí.

Dr. Ortiz: ¿Cuándo está deprimida le da por comer?

Amalia: Sí, me da por comer.

Dr. Ortiz: ¿Y está muy nerviosa por muchas cosas?

[00:26:29]   ¿Tiene la cabeza así como que piense, piense y piense y piense o sólo en las noches cuando no puede dormir?

Amalia: No. No, es una [inaudible] en las noches y pues estoy como mal porque me siento que es como que resalto y resalto. Digo, pues no tiene caso pero según yo.

Dr. Ortiz: Pues si sirve, ¿no?

Amalia: Pues yo pienso que sí porque de menos—

[Fin del audio]

Duración: 27 minutos

REFERENCES

Ainsworth-Vaughn, Nancy. 1998. *Claiming Power in Doctor–Patient Talk*. New York: Oxford University Press.

Alegría, Margarita, Pinka Chatterji, Kenneth Wells, Zhun Cao, Chih-nan Chen, David Takeuchi, James Jackson, and Xiao-Li Meng. 2008. "Disparity in Depression Treatment among Racial and Ethnic Minority Populations in the United States." *Psychiatric Services* 59, no. 11: 1264–72.

Allison, Abigail, and Karol Hardin. 2020. "Missed Opportunities to Build Rapport: A Pragmalinguistic Analysis of Interpreted Medical Conversations with Spanish-Speaking Patients." *Health Communication* 35, no. 4: 494–501.

Altarriba, Jeanette, and Azara L. Santiago-Rivera. 1994. "Current Perspectives on Using Linguistic and Cultural Factors in Counseling the Hispanic Client." *Professional Psychology: Research and Practice* 25, no 4: 388–97.

American Psychiatric Association. 2017. "Mental Health Disparities: Hispanics and Latinos." https://www.psychiatry.org/File%20Library/Psychiatrists/Cultural-Competency/Mental-Health-Disparities/Mental-Health-Facts-for-Hispanic-Latino.pdf.

Andrews, Jane, Richard Fay, and Ross White. 2018. "What Shapes Everyday Translanguaging? Insights from a Global Mental Health Project in Northern Uganda." In *Translanguaging as Everyday Practice,* edited by Geraldo Mazzaferro, 257–73. New York: Springer Berlin Heidelberg. https://doi.org/10.1007/978-3-319-94851-5_14.

Añez, Luis M., Manuel París Jr., Luis E. Bedregal, Larry Davidson, and Carlos M. Grilo. 2005. "Application of Cultural Constructs in the Care of First-Generation Latino Clients in a Community Mental Health Setting." *Journal of Psychiatric Practice* 11, no. 4: 221–30.

Angelelli, Claudia. 2004. *Medical Interpreting and Cross-Cultural Communication*. Cambridge: Cambridge University Press.

Angermeyer, Philipp Sebastian. 2010. "Interpreter-Mediated Interaction as Bilingual Speech: Bridging Macro- and Micro-Sociolinguistics in Codeswitching Research." *International Journal of Bilingualism* 14, no. 4: 466–89. https://doi.org/10.1177/1367006910370914.

Antshel, Kevin M. 2002. "Integrating Culture as a Means of Improving Treatment Adherence in the Latino Population." *Psychology, Health and Medicine* 7, no. 4: 435–49. https://doi.org/10.1080/1354850021000015258.

Association of American Medical Colleges. 2016. "Diversity in Medical Education: Facts and Figures: Current Trends in Medical Education." http://www.aamcdiversityfactsandfigures2016.org/report-section/section-3/.

Barr, Donald A., and Stanley F. Wanat. 2005. "Listening to Patients: Cultural and Linguistic Barriers to Health Care Access." *Family Medicine* 37, no. 3: 199–204.

Bauer, Amy M., Chih-Nan Chen, and Margarita Alegría. 2010. "English Language Proficiency and Mental Health Service use Among Latino and Asian Americans with Mental Disorders." *Medical Care* 48, no. 12: 1097–104.

Betancourt, Hector, Patricia M. Flynn, and Sarah R. Ormseth. 2011. "Healthcare Mistreatment and Continuity of Cancer Screening among Latino and Anglo American Women in Southern California." *Women and Health* 51, no. 1: 1–24. http://dx.doi.org/10.1080/03630242.2011.541853.

Blanchard, Janice, and Nicole Lurie. 2004. "R-E-S-P-E-C-T: Patient Reports of Disrespect in the Health Care Setting and Its Impact on Care." *The Journal of Family Practice* 53, no. 9: 721–30.

Bloom, Rachel. 2014. "Negotiating Language in Transnational Health Care: Exploring Translingual Literacy through Grounded Practical Theory." *Journal of Applied Communication Research* 42, no. 3: 268–84.

Bloom-Pojar, Rachel. 2018. *Translanguaging Outside the Academy: Negotiating Rhetoric and Healthcare in the Spanish Caribbean.* Urbana, IL: National Council of Teachers of English.

Brenneisen-Goode, Mercedes. 2008. "We Talked About Our Lives, Our Dreams, Our Disappointments." In *The Art of Healing Latinos: Firsthand Accounts from Physicians and Other Health Advocates,* 2nd ed., edited by David E. Hayes-Bautista and Roberto Chiprut, 80–90. Los Angeles: UCLA Chicano Studies Research Center Press.

Brown, Penelope, and Stephen C. Levinson. 1987. *Politeness: Some Universals in Language Usage.* Cambridge: Cambridge University Press.

Caballero, A. Enrique. 2011. "Understanding the Hispanic/Latino Patient." *The American Journal of Medicine* 124, no. 10: S10–S15. https://doi.org/10.1016/j.amjmed.2011.07.018.

Cabassa, Leopoldo J., Marissa C. Hansen, Lawrence A. Palinkas, and Kathleen Ell. 2008. "Azúcar y Nervios: Explanatory Models and Treatment Experiences of Hispanics with Diabetes and Depression." *Social Science and Medicine* 66, no. 12: 2413–24.

Caffi, Claudia. 1999. "On Mitigation." *Journal of Pragmatics* 31, no. 7: 881–909.

Caffi, Claudia. 2007. *Mitigation.* Amsterdam: Elsevier.

Carlat, Daniel J. 2012. *The Psychiatric Interview,* 3rd ed. Philadelphia: Lippincott William and Wilkins.

Carreira, María, and Olga Kagan. 2011. "The Results of the National Heritage Language Survey: Implications for Teaching, Curriculum Design, and Professional Development." *Foreign Language Annals* 44, no. 1: 40–64.

Charteris-Black, Jonathan. 2012. "Shattering the Bell Jar: Metaphor, Gender, and Depression." *Metaphor and Symbol* 27, no. 3: 199–216.

CHIA Standards and Certification Committee. 2002. *California Standards for Health-Care Interpreters: Ethical Principles, Protocols, and Guidance on Roles and Intervention.* Sacramento: California Endowment.

Colombi, María Cecilia. 2003. "Un Enfoque Funcional para la Enseñanza del Lenguaje Expositivo." In *Mi Lengua: Spanish as a Heritage Language in the United States, Research and Practice,* edited by Ana Roca and Cecilia Colombi, 78–95. Washington, DC: Georgetown University Press.

Colombi, María Cecilia, and Dalia Magaña. 2013. "Alfabetización Avanzada en Español en los Estados Unidos en el siglo XXI." In *El Español en los Estados Unidos: E Pluribus Unum? Enfoques multidisciplinarios,* edited by Domnita Dumitrescu and Gerardo Piña-Rosales, 339–52. New York: Academia Norteamericana de la Lengua Española.

Colon, Eduardo, Aida Giachello, LaShawn McIver, Guadalupe Pacheco, and Leonel Vela. 2013. "Diabetes and Depression in the Hispanic/Latino community." *Clinical Diabetes* 31, no. 1: 43–45.

Cordella, Marisa. 2000. "Medical Discourse in a Hispanic Environment: Power and Simpatía under Examination." *Australian Review of Applied Linguistics* 22, no. 2: 35–50.

Cordella, Marisa. 2004. *The Dynamic Consultation: A Discourse Analytical Study of Doctor-Patient Communication.* Amsterdam/Philadelphia: John Benjamins.

Cordella, Marisa. 2007. "'No, no I haven't been taking it doctor': Noncompliance, Face Threatening Acts and Politeness in Medical Consultations." In *Research on Politeness in the Spanish-Speaking World,* edited by Marie Elena Placencia and Carmen Garcia, 191–212. Mahwah, NJ: Lawrence Erlbaum.

Coupland, Justine. 2000. "Introduction: Sociolinguistic Perspectives on Small Talk." In *Small Talk,* edited by Justine Coupland, 1–25. Harlow, UK: Pearson Education.

Curcó, Carmen. 1998. "¿No me harías un favorcito? Reflexiones en Torno a la Expresión de la Cortesía Verbal en el español de México y el español Peninsular." In *La Pragmática Lingüística del español: Recientes Desarrollos, Diálogos Hispánicos,* edited by Henk Haverkate, Gijs Mulder, and Caroline Fraile Maldonado, Diálogos hispánicos 22, 129–72.

Davidson, Brad. 1997. "Diagnosing Illness Across Languages: The Role of Interpreters in Medical Discourse." *Proceedings of the Twenty-Third Annual Meeting of the Berkeley Linguistics Society: General Session and Parasession on Pragmatics and Grammatical Structure* 23, no. 1: 62–71.

Davidson, Brad. 2000. "The Interpreter as Institutional Gatekeeper: The Social-Linguistic Role of Interpreter in Spanish-English Medical Discourse." *Journal of Sociolinguistics* 4, no. 3: 379–405.

Davidson, Brad. 2001. "Questions in Cross-Linguistic Medical Encounter: The Role of the Hospital Interpreter." *Anthropological Quarterly* 74, no. 4: 170–78.

Davis, Kia L., Mary O'Toole, Carol A. Brownson, Patricia Llanos, and Edwin B. Fisher. 2007. "Teaching How, Not What: The Contributions of Community Health Workers to Diabetes Self-Management." *The Diabetes Educator* 33, no. 6: 208S–215S.

De la Torre, Adela, and Antonio L. Estrada. 2015. *Mexican Americans and Health: Sana! Sana!,* 2nd ed. Tucson: University of Arizona Press.

De Silva Joyce, Helen, Diana Slade, Deborah Bateson, Hermine Scheeres, Jeannette McGregor, and Edith Weisberg. 2015. "Patient-Centered Discourse in Sexual and Reproductive Health Consultations." *Discourse and Communication* 9, no. 3: 275–92. https://doi.org/10.1177/1750481315571162.

Deeb-Sossa, Natalia, ed. 2019. *Community-Based Participatory Research: Testimonios from Chicana/o Studies.* Tucson: University of Arizona Press. https://doi.org/10.2307/j.ctvdjrpp5.

Delbene, Roxana. 2004. "The Function of Mitigation in the Context of a Socially Stigmatized Disease: A Case Study in a Public Hospital in Montevideo, Uruguay." *Spanish in Context* 1, no. 2: 241–67.

Dingfelder, Sadie. 2005. "Closing the Gap for Latino Patients." *Monitor on Psychology* 36, no. 1: 58–61. https://www.apa.org/monitor/jan05/closingthegap.aspx.

Eamranond, Pracha, Roger B. Davis, Russell S. Phillips, and Christina C. Wee. 2009. "Patient-Physician Language Concordance and Lifestyle Counseling among Spanish-Speaking Patients." *Journal of Immigrant Minority Health* 11, no. 6: 494–98.

Eggins, Suzanne. 2004. *An Introduction to Systemic Functional Linguistics,* 2nd ed. London: Continuum.

Eggins, Suzanne, and Diana Slade. 2005. *Analyzing Casual Conversation.* London: Cassell.

Eggly, Susan. 2002. "Physician-Patient Co-construction of Illness Narratives in the Medical Interview." *Health Communication* 14, no. 3: 339–60.

Eggly Susan, Felicity W. Harper, Louis A. Penner, Marci J. Gleason, Tanina Foster, and Terrance L. Albrecht. 2011. "Variation in Question Asking during Cancer Clinical Interactions: A Potential Source of Disparities in Access to Information." *Patient Education and Counseling* 82, no. 1: 63–68.

Elderkin-Thompson, Virginia, Roxanne Cohen Silver, and Howard Waitzkin. 2001. "When Nurses Double as Interpreters: A Study of Spanish-Speaking Patients in a U.S. Primary Care Setting." *Social Science and Medicine* 52, no. 9: 1343–58.

Elías-Olivares, Lucía. 1976. "Ways of Speaking in a Chicano Community: A Socio-Linguistic Approach." PhD diss., University of Texas at Austin.

Erzinger, Sharry. 1991. "Communication between Spanish-Speaking Patients and Their Doctors in Medical Encounters." *Culture, Medicine, Psychiatry* 15, no. 1: 91–110.

Fernandez, Alicia, Dean Schillinger, E. Margaret Warton, Nancy Adler, Howard H. Moffet, Yael Schenker, M. Victoria Salgado, Ameena Ahmed, and Andrew J. Karter. 2011. "Language Barriers, Physician-Patient Language Concordance, and Glycemic Control among Insured Latinos with Diabetes: The Diabetes Study of Northern California (DISTANCE)." *Journal of General Internal Medicine* 26, no. 2: 170–76. https://doi.org/10.1007/s11606-010-1507-6.

Ferrara, Kathleen Warden. 1994. *Therapeutic Ways with Words.* New York: Oxford University Press.

Figueras Bates, Carolina. 2020. "Cognitive and Affective Dimensions of Mitigation in Advice." *Corpus Pragmatics* 4, no. 1: 31–57. https://doi.org/10.1007/s41701-019-00064-x.

First, Michael B., Miriam Gibbon, Robert L. Spitzer, Lorna Smith Benjamin, and Janet B. W. Williams. 1997. *Structured Clinical Interview for DSM-IV Axis II Personality Disorders: SCID-II.* Washington, DC: American Psychiatric Press.

Flores, Glenn. 2000. "Culture and the Patient-Physician Relationship: Achieving Cultural Competency in Health Care." *The Journal of Pediatrics* 136, no. 1: 14–23. https://doi.org/10.1016/S0022-3476(00)90043-X.

Flores, Glenn. 2006. "Language Barriers to Health Care in the United States." *New England Journal of Medicine* 355, no. 3: 229–31.

Flores, Yvette G. 2013. *Chicana and Chicano Mental Health: Alma, Mente y Corazón.* Tucson: University of Arizona Press.

Flores-Ferrán, Nydia. 2010 "An Examination of Mitigation Strategies Used in Spanish Psychotherapeutic Discourse." *Journal of Pragmatics* 42, no. 7: 1964–81.

Flores-Ferrán, Nydia. 2012. "Pragmatic Variation in Therapeutic Discourse: An Examination of Mitigating Devices Employed by Dominican Female Clients and a Cuban American Therapist." In *Pragmatic Variation in First and Second Language Contexts: Methodological Issues,* edited by J. César Félix-Brasdefer and Dale A. Koike, 81–112. Philadelphia: John Benjamins.

Flynn, Patricia M., Hector Betancourt, Carlos Garberoglio, Gregory J. Regts, Kayla M. Kinworthy, and Daniel J. Northington. 2015. "Attributions and Emotions Regarding Health Care Mistreatment Impact Continuity of Care among Latino and Anglo American Women." *Cultural Diversity and Ethnic Minority Psychology* 21, no. 4: 593–603. https://doi.org/10.1037/cdp0000019.

Frankel, Richard. 1990. "Talking in Interviews: A Dispreference for Patient-Initiated Questions in Physician–Patient Encounters." In *Everyday Language: Studies in Ethnomethodology,* edited by George Psathas, 231–62. New York: Irvington.

Fraser, Bruce. 1980. "Conversational Mitigation." *Journal of Pragmatics* 4, no. 4: 341–50.

Fung, Loretta, and Ronald Carter. 2007. "Discourse Markers and Spoken English: Native and Learner Use in Pedagogic Settings." *Applied Linguistics* 28, no. 3: 410–39. https://doi.org/10.1093/applin/amm030.

Garachana Camarero, Mar. 2008. "Cuestiones Pragmáticas sobre la Negación." *Revista Electrónica de Didáctica ELE* 5, no. 12.

García, Caroline Marie, Lauren Gilchrist, Gabriela Vazquez, Amy Leite, and Nancy Raymond. 2011. "Urban and Rural Immigrant Latino Youths' and Adults' Knowledge and Beliefs about Mental Health Resources." *Journal of Immigrant and Minority Health* 13, no. 3: 500–509. https://doi.org/10.1007/s10903-010-9389-6.

García, Ofelia. 2009. *Bilingual Education in the 21st Century: A Global Perspective.* Malden, MA: Wiley-Blackwell.

García, Ofelia, and Li Wei. 2014. *Translanguaging: Language, Bilingualism and Education.* New York: Palgrave Macmillan.

Geisler, Michael, Claire Kramsch, Scott McGinnis, Peter Patrikis, Mary Louis Pratt, Karin Ryding, Haun Saussy. 2007. "Foreign Languages and Higher Education: New Structures for a Changed World: MLA Ad Hoc Committee on Foreign Languages." *Profession* 2007: 234–45.

Guarnaccia, Peter J., Victor DeLaCancela, and Emilio Carrillo. 1989. "The Multiple Meanings of Ataques de Nervios in the Latino Community." *Medical Anthropology* 11, no. 1: 47–62. https://doi.org/10.1080/01459740.1989.9965981.

Gumperz, John. 1982. *Discourse Strategies.* Cambridge: Cambridge University Press.

Halliday, Michael A. K. 1978. *Language as Social Semiotic: The Social Interpretation of Language and Meaning.* London: Edward Arnold.

Halliday, Michael A. K., and Christian M. I. M. Matthiessen. 2004. *An Introduction to Functional Grammar,* 3rd ed. London: Edward Arnold.

Hansen, Marissa C., and Leopoldo J. Cabassa. 2012. "Pathways to Depression Care: Help-Seeking Experiences of Low-Income Latinos with Diabetes and Depression." *Journal of Immigrant and Minority Health* 14, no. 6: 1097–106.

Hardin, Karol. 2012. "Targeting Oral and Cultural Proficiency for Medical Personnel: An Examination of Current Medical Spanish Textbooks." *Hispania* 95, no. 4: 698–713.

Hayes-Bautista, David E., and Robert Chiprut. 2008. *The Art of Healing Latinos: Firsthand Accounts from Physicians and Other Health Advocates,* 2nd ed. Los Angeles: UCLA Chicano Studies Research Center Press.

Hernández, Claudia, Mayra Cruz, and June K. Robinson. 2011. "Spanish-Speaking Patient Health Educational Preferences." *Archives of Dermatology* 147, no. 2: 242–44. https://doi.org/10.1001/archdermatol.2010.421

Holmes, Janet. 1986. "Functions of *you know* in Women's and Men's Speech." *Language in Society* 15, no. 1: 1–21.

Hyland, Ken. 1996. "Writing without Conviction? Hedging in Science Research Articles." *Applied Linguistics* 17, no. 4: 433–54.

Ingram, Maia, Emma Torres, Flor Redondo, Gail Bradford, Chin Wang, and Mary L. O'Toole. 2007. "The Impact of *Promotoras* on Social Support and Glycemic Control among Members of a Farmworker Community on the US-Mexico Border." *Diabetes Educator* 33, no. 6: 172S–178S.

Interian, Alejandro, Alonso Ang, Michael A. Gara, Michael A. Rodriguez, and William A. Vega. 2011. "The Long-Term Trajectory of Depression among Latinos in Primary Care and Its Relationship to Depression Care Disparities." *General Hospital Psychiatry* 33, no. 2: 94–101.

Jacobson, Rodolfo. 1982. "The Social Implications of Intra-sentential Code-Switching." In *Spanish in the United States: Sociolinguistics Aspects,* edited by Jon Amastae and Lucía Elías-Olivares, 182–208. Cambridge: Cambridge University Press.

Josephson, Irene, Robyn Woodward-Kron, Clare Delany, and Amy Hiller. 2015. "Evaluative Language in Physiotherapy Practice: How Does It Contribute to the Therapeutic Relationship?" *Social Science and Medicine* 143: 128–36.

Joshu, Corinne E., Lourdes Rangel, Otila Garcia, Carol A. Brownson, and Mary L. O'Toole. 2007. "Integration of a Promotora-Led Self-Management Program into a System of Care." *The Diabetes Educator* 33, no. 6: 151S–158S.

Juckett, Gregory. 2013. "Caring for Latino Patients." *American Family Physician* 87, no. 1: 48–54.

Katz, Marra G., Terry A. Jacobson, Emir Veledar, and Sunil Kripalani. 2007. "Patient Literacy and Question-Asking Behavior during the Medical Encounter: A Mixed-Methods Analysis." *Journal of General Internal Medicine* 22, no. 6: 782–86.

Koike, Dale April. 1994. "Negation in Spanish and English Suggestions and Requests: Mitigating Effects?" *Journal of Pragmatics* 21, no. 5: 513–26. https://doi.org/10.1016/0378-2166(94)90027-2.

Kramsch, Claire. 2010. "Theorizing Translingual/Transcultural Competence." In *Critical and Intercultural Theory and Language Pedagogy,* edited by Glenn S. Levine and Alison M. Phipps, 15–31. Boston: Heinle Cengage Learning.

Labov, William, and David Fanshel. 1977. *Therapeutic Discourse: Psychotherapy as Conversation.* New York: Academic Press.

Labov, William, and Joshua Waletzky. 1997. "Narrative Analysis: Oral Versions of Personal Experience." *Journal of Narrative & Life History* 7, nos. 1–4: 3–38. https://doi.org/10.1075/jnlh.7.02nar.

Lackey, Gerald F. 2008. "'Feeling Blue' in Spanish: A Qualitative Inquiry of Depression among Mexican Immigrants." *Social Science and Medicine* 67, no. 2: 228–37.

Lee, Linda J., Holly A. Batal, Judith H. Maselli, and Jean S. Kutner. 2002. "Effect of Spanish Interpretation Method on Patient Satisfaction in an Urban Walk-In Clinic." *Journal General Internal Medicine* 17, no. 8: 641–46.

Lin, Luona, Andrew Nigrinis, Peggy Christidis, and Karen Stamm. 2015. *Demographics of the US Psychology Workforce: Findings from the American Community Survey.* Washington, DC: American Psychological Association Center for Workforce Studies. http://www.apa.org/workforce/publications/13-demographics/index.aspx.

López, Alberto G., and Ernestina Carrillo, eds. 2001. *The Latino Psychiatric Patient: Assessment and Treatment.* Washington, DC, and London: American Psychiatric Publishing.

López, Alberto, and Israel Katz. 2001. "An Introduction to Latinos in the United States." In *The Latino Psychiatric Patient: Assessment and Treatment,* edited by Alberto López and Ernestina Carrillo, 3–17. Washington, DC: American Psychiatric Publishing.

López-Cevallos, Daniel F., S. Marie Harvey, and Jocelyn T. Warren. 2014. "Medical Mistrust, Perceived Discrimination, and Satisfaction with Health Care among Young-Adult Rural Latinos." *The Journal of Rural Health* 30, no. 4: 344–51.

Magaña, Dalia. 2016. "Code-Switching in Social-Network Messages: A Case Study of a Bilingual Chicana." *International Journal of the Linguistic Association of the Southwest* (2013) 32, no. 1: 43–65.

Magaña, Dalia. 2017. "Modality Resources in Spanish during Psychiatric Interviews with Mexican Patients." *Communication and Medicine* 13, no. 3: 291–305.

Magaña, Dalia. 2018a. "*Órale, ¿cómo le haces?*: Small Talk Genres during the Psychiatric Interview in Spanish." *International Journal of the Linguistic Association of the Southwest* (2014), 33, no. 1: 75–96.

Magaña, Dalia. 2018b. "Code-Switching." In *An Introduction to Bilingualism: Principles and Processes (2nd edition),* edited by Jeanette Altarriba and Roberto R. Heredia, 317–32. New York: Taylor and Francis Group.

Magaña, Dalia. 2019. "Cultural Competence and Metaphor in Mental Healthcare Interactions: A Linguistic Perspective." *Patient Education & Counseling,* 102, no. 12: 2192–98.

Magaña, Dalia. 2020. "Local Voices on Health Care Communication Issues and Insights on Latino Cultural Constructs." *Hispanic Journal of Behavioral Sciences* 42, no. 3: 300–323.

Marquez, Jorge A., and Jorge I. Ramírez García. 2013. "Family Caregivers' Narratives of Mental Health Treatment Usage Processes by their Latino Adult Relatives with Serious and Persistent Mental Illness." *Journal of Family Psychology* 27, no. 3: 398–408. https://doi.org/10.1037/a0032868.

Martin, James R., and David Rose. 2007. *Working with Discourse,* 2nd ed. London: Continuum.

Martin, James R., and David Rose. 2008. *Genre Relations: Mapping Culture.* London: Equinox.

Martin, James R., and Peter White. 2005. *The Language of Evaluation: Appraisal in English.* New York: Palgrave Macmillan.

Martínez, Glenn A. 2003. "Classroom Based Dialect Awareness in Heritage Language Instruction: A Critical Applied Linguistic Approach." *Heritage Language Journal* 1, no. 1: 1–14.

Martínez, Glenn A. 2008. "Language-in-Healthcare Policy, Interaction Patterns, and Unequal Care on the U.S.-Mexico Border." *Language Policy* 7, no. 4: 345–63.

Martínez, Glenn A. 2010. "Medical Spanish for Heritage Learners: A Prescription to Improve the Health of Spanish-Speaking Communities." In *Building Communities and Making Connections,* edited by Susana Rivera-Mills and Juan Antonio Trujillo, 2–15. Newcastle upon Tyne: Cambridge Scholars.

Martínez, Glenn A. 2011. "Language and Power in Healthcare: Towards a Theory of Language Barriers Among Linguistic Minorities in the United States." In *Readings in Language Studies,* vol. 2, *Language and Power,* edited by John Louis Watzke, Paul Chamness Miller and Miguel Mantero, 59–74. Saint Louis: International Society for Language Studies.

Martínez, Glenn A., and Adam Schwartz. 2012. "Elevating 'Low' Language for High Stakes: A Case for Critical, Community-Based Learning in a Medical Spanish for Heritage Learners Program." *Heritage Language Journal* 9, no. 2: 37–49.

Matthiessen, Christian M. I. M. 2013. "Applying Systemic Functional Linguistics in Healthcare Contexts." *Text and Talk* 33, no. 4–5: 437–66.

Maynard, Douglas W., and Pamela L. Hudak. 2008. "Small Talk, High Stakes: Interactional Disattentiveness in the Context of Prosocial Doctor-Patient Interaction." *Language in Society* 37, no. 5: 661–88.

McDonald, Daniel, and Robyn Woodward-Kron. 2016. "Member Roles and Identities in Online Support Groups: Perspectives from Corpus and Systemic Functional Linguistics." *Discourse and Communication* 10, no. 2: 157–75. https://doi.org/10.1177/1750481315615985.

McEwen, Marylyn Morris, Alice Pasgovel, Gwen Gallegos, and Lourdes Barrera. 2010. "Type 2 Diabetes Self-Management Social Support Intervention at the U.S.-Mexico Border." *Public Health Nursing* 27, no. 4: 310–19.

McGuire, Allison A., Isabel C. Garcés-Palacio, and Isabel C. Scarinci. 2012. "A Successful Guide in Understanding Latino Immigrant Patients: An Aid for Health Care Professionals." *Family and Community Health* 35, no. 1: 76–84. https://doi.org/10.1097/FCH.0b013e3182385d7c.

McMullen, Linda M., and John B. Conway. 2002. "Conventional Metaphors for Depression." In *The Verbal Communication of Emotions,* edited by Susan R. Fussell, 167–81. New York: Psychology Press.

Menendez, Mariano E., Bastiaan T. Van Hoorn, Michael Mackert, Erin E. Donovan, Neal C. Chen, and David Ring. 2017. "Patients with Limited Health Literacy Ask Fewer Questions during Office Visits with Hand Surgeons." *Clinical Orthopaedics and Related Research* 475, no. 5: 1291–97. https://doi.org/10.1007/s11999-016-5140-5.

Mihatsch, Wiltrud. 2009. "The Approximators French *comme,* Italian *come,* Portuguese *como* and Spanish *como* from a Grammaticalization Perspective." In *Grammaticalization and Pragmatics: Facts, Approaches, Theoretical Issues,* edited by Corinne Rossari, Claudia Ricci, and Adriana Spiridon, 65–91. Leiden: Brill.

Mishler, Elliot. 1984. *The Discourse of Medicine: Dialectics of Medical Interviews.* Norwood, NJ: Ablex.

Musanti, Sandra I., and Alma D. Rodríguez. 2017. "Translanguaging in Bilingual Teacher Preparation: Exploring Pre-Service Bilingual Teachers' Academic Writing." *Bilingual Research Journal* 40, no. 1: 38–54. https://doi.org/10.1080/15235882.2016.1276028.

Nadeem, Erum, Jane M. Lange, Dawn Edge, Marie Fongwa, Tom Belin, and Jeanne Miranda. 2007. "Does Stigma Keep Poor Young Immigrant and US-Born Black and Latina Women from Seeking Mental Health Care?" *Psychiatric Services* 58, no. 12: 1547–54.

Ngo-Metzger, Quyen, Dara H. Sorkin, Russell S. Phillips, Sheldon Greenfield, Michael P. Massagli, Brain Clarridge, and Sherrie H. Kaplan. 2007. "Providing High-Quality Care for Limited English Proficient Patients: The Importance of Language Concordance and Interpreter Use." *Journal of General Internal Medicine* 22, no. 2: 324–30. https://doi.org/10.1007/s11606-007-0340-z.

Nieves-Ruiz, Randy. 2010. "Language a Barrier to Health Care." *Newsweek,* June 9, 2010, http://www.newsweek.com/language-barrier-health-care-73335.

Nightingale, Richard, and Pilar Safont. 2019. "Pragmatic Translanguaging: Multilingual Practice in Adolescent Online Discourse." In *Investigating the Learning of Pragmatics across Ages and Contexts,* edited by Patricia Salazar-Campillo and Victòria Codina-Espurz, 167–95. Boston: Brill Rodopi. https://doi.org/10.1163/9789004409699_009.

Odor, Alberto, Peter Yellowlees, Donald Hilty, Michelle Burke Parish, Najia Nafiz, and Ana-Maria Iosif. 2011. "PsychVACS: A System for Asynchronous Telepsychiatry." *Telemedicine and e-Health* 17, no. 4: 299–303.

Office of Minority Health. 2013. *National Standards for Culturally and Linguistically Appropriate Services in Health and Health Care.* Washington, DC: US Department of Health and Human Services. https://thinkculturalhealth.hhs.gov/assets/pdfs/EnhancedCLASStandardsBlueprint.pdf

Ortega, Pilar. 2018. "Spanish Language Concordance in U.S. Medical Care: A Multifaceted Challenge and Call to Action." *Academic Medicine: Journal of the Association of American Medical Colleges* 93, no. 9: 1276–80. https://doi.org/10.1097/ACM.0000000000002307.

Ortega, Pilar, Lisa Diamond, Marco A. Alemán, Jaime Fatás-Cabeza, Dalia Magaña, Valarie Pazo, Norma Pérez, Jorge A. Girotti, Elena Ríos, and Medical Spanish Summit. 2020. "Medical Spanish Standardization in U.S. Medical Schools: Consensus Statement from a Multidisciplinary Expert Panel." *Academic Medicine: Journal of the Association of American Medical Colleges* 95, no. 1: 22–31. https://doi.org/10.1097/ACM.0000000000002917.

Ortega, Pilar, and Josh Prada. 2020. "Words Matter: Translanguaging in Medical Communication Skills Training." *Perspectives on Medical Education* 9: 251–55. https://doi.org/10.1007/s40037-020-00595-z.

Otheguy, Ricardo, Ofelia García, and Wallis Reid. 2015. "Clarifying Translanguaging and Deconstructing Named Languages: A Perspective from Linguistics." *Applied Linguistics Review* 6, no. 3: 281–307. https://doi.org/10.1515/applirev-2015-0014.

Palmer, Deborah K., Ramón Antonio Martínez, Suzanne G. Mateus, and Kathryn Henderson. 2014. "Reframing the Debate on Language Separation: Toward a Vision for Translanguaging Pedagogies in the Dual Language Classroom." *The Modern Language Journal* 98, no. 3: 757–72. https://doi.org/10.1111/modl.12121.

Perez-Stable, Eliseo J., Anna Nápoles-Springer, and José M. Miramontes. 1997. "The Effects of Ethnicity and Language on Medical Outcomes of Patients with Hypertension or Diabetes." *Medical Care* 35, no. 12: 1212–19.

Poplack, Shana. 1982. "Sometimes I'll Start a Sentence in Spanish y Termino en español: Toward a Typology of Code-Switching." In *Spanish in the United States: Sociolinguistics Aspects,* edited by Jon Amastae and Lucía Elías-Olivares, 230–63. Cambridge: Cambridge University Press.

Poynton, Cate. 1989. *Language and Gender: Making the Difference.* Oxford: Oxford University Press.

Poza, Luis E. 2019. "'*Los Dos Son Mi Idioma*': Translanguaging, Identity, and Social Relationships among Bilingual Youth." *Journal of Language, Identity and Education* 18, no. 2: 92–109. https://doi.org/10.1080/15348458.2018.1504682.

Pratt, Laura A., Debra J. Brody, and Qiuping Gu. 2011. "Antidepressant Use in Persons Aged 12 and Over: United States, 2005–2008." *NCHS Data Brief* 76 (October): 1–8.

Ragan, Sandy L. 2000. "Sociable Talk in Women's Health Care Contexts: Two Forms of Non-Medical Talk." In *Small Talk,* edited by Justine Coupland, 269–87. Harlow, UK: Pearson Education. https://doi.org/10.4324/9781315838328-15.

Raymond, Chase Wesley. 2014a. "Conveying Information in the Interpreter-Mediated Medical Visit: The Case of Epistemic Brokering." *Patient Education and Counseling* 97, no. 1: 38–46.

Raymond, Chase Wesley. 2014b. "Epistemic Brokering in the Interpreter-Mediated Medical Visit: Negotiating 'Patient's Side' and 'Doctor's Side' Knowledge." *Research on Language and Social Interaction* 47, no. 4: 426–46.

Raymond-Flesch, Marissa, Rachel Siemons, Nadereh Pourat, Ken Jacobs, and Claire D. Brindis. 2014. "'There Is No Help Out There and If There Is, It's Really Hard to Find': A Qualitative Study of the Health Concerns and Health Care Access of Latino 'DREAMers.'" *Journal of Adolescent Health* 55, no. 3: 323–28.

Rastogi, Mudita, Nicole Massey-Hastings, and Elizabeth Wieling. 2012. "Barriers to Seeking Mental Health Services in the Latino/a Community: A Qualitative Analysis." *Journal of Systemic Therapies* 31, no. 4: 1–17. https://doi.org/10.1521/jsyt.2012.31.4.1.

Real Academia Española. 2014. *Diccionario de la Lengua Española,* 23rd ed. Madrid: Espasa Calpe. http://lema.rae.es/drae/?val=spanglish.

Roberts, Celia, and Srikant Sarangi. 2005. "Theme-Oriented Discourse Analysis of Medical Encounters." *Medical Education* 39, no. 6: 632–40.

Sánchez-Muñoz, Ana. 2007. "Style Variation in Spanish as a Heritage Language: A Study of Discourse Particles in Academic and Non-academic Registers." In *Spanish in Contact: Policy, Social and Linguistic Inquiries,* edited by Kim Potowski and Richard Cameron, 153–71. New York: John Benjamins.

Santiago-Rivera, Azara L., and Jeanette Altarriba. 2002. "The Role of Language in Therapy with the Spanish-English Bilingual Client." *Professional Psychology: Research and Practice,* 33, no. 1: 30–38. https://doi.org/10.1037/0735-7028.33.1.30.

Sentell, Tetine, and Kathryn L. Braun. 2012. "Low Health Literacy, Limited English Proficiency, and Health Status in Asians, Latinos, and Other Racial/Ethnic Groups in California." *Journal of Health Communication: International Perspectives* 17, no. 3: 82–99.

Sentell, Tetine, Martha Shumway, and Lonnie Snowden. 2007. "Access to Mental Health Treatment by English Language Proficiency and Race/Ethnicity." *Journal of General Internal Medicine* 22, no. 2: 289–93.

Shea, Shawn Cristopher. 1998. *Psychiatric Interviewing: The Art of Understanding: A Practical Guide for Psychiatrists, Psychologists, Counselors, Social Workers, Nurses, and Other Mental Health Professionals,* 2nd ed. Philadelphia: W. B. Saunders.

Sheehan, David V., Yves Lecrubier, K. Harnett Sheehan, Patricia Amorim, Juris Janavs, Emmanuelle Weiller, Thierry Hergueta, Roxy Baker, and Geoffrey C. Dunbar. 1998. "The Mini-International Neuropsychiatric Interview (MINI): The Development and Validation of a Structured Diagnostic Psychiatric Interview for DSM-IV and ICD-10." *The Journal of Clinical Psychiatry* 59, Suppl. 20: 22–57.

Slade, Diana, Hermine Scheeres, Marie Manidis, Rick Iedema, Roger Dunston, Jane Stein-Parbury, Christian Matthiessen, María Herke, and Jeannette McGregor. 2008. "Emergency Communication: The Discursive Challenges Facing Emergency Clinicians and Patients in Hospital Emergency Departments." *Discourse and Communication* 2, no. 3: 271–98.

Stivers, Tanya. 2007. *Prescribing Under Pressure: Parent-Physician Conversations and Antibiotics.* New York: Oxford University Press.

Stivers, Tanya, and John Heritage. 2001. "Breaking the Sequential Mold: Answering 'More than the Question' during Comprehensive History Taking." *Text and Talk* 21, no 1–2: 151–85.

Tagliamonte, Sali. 2005. "*So* Who? *Like* How? *Just* What? Discourse Markers in the Conversations of Young Canadians." *Journal of Pragmatics* 37, no. 11: 1896–915.

Tardy, Christine M. 2011. "Genre Analysis." In *Bloomsbury Companion to Discourse Analysis,* edited by Ken Hyland and Brian Paltridge, 54–68. London: Continuum.

Tebble, Helen. 2008. "Using SFL to Understand and Practise Dialogue Interpreting." In *Proceedings of ISFC 35: Voices around the World,* edited by Canzhong Wu, Christian M. I. M. Matthiessen, and Marie Herke, 146–51. Sydney, NSW: 35th ISFC Organizing Committee.

ten Have, Paul. 1991. "Talk and Institution: A Reconsideration of the 'Asymmetry' of Doctor-Patient Interaction." In *Talk and Social Structure: Studies in Ethnomethodology and Conversation Analysis,* edited by Deirdre Boden and Don H. Zimmerman, 138–63. Cambridge: Polity Press.

Timmins, Caraway. 2002. "The Impact of Language Barriers on the Health Care of Latinos in the United States: A Review of the Literature and Guidelines for Practice." *Journal of Midwifery and Women's Health* 47, no. 2: 80–96.

Toribio, Almeida Jacqueline. 2000. "Spanglish?! Bite Your Tongue! Spanish-English Code-Switching among Latinos." In *Reflexiones 1999: New Directions in Mexican American Studies*, edited by Richard R. Flores, 115–47. Austin, TX: Center for Mexican American Studies.

Uebelacker, Lisa A., Beth A. Marootian, Paul A. Pirraglia, Jennifer Primack, Patrick M. Tigue, Ryan Haggarty, Lavina Velazquez, Jennifer J. Bowdoin, Zornitsa Kalibatseva, and Ivan W. Miller. 2012. "Barriers and Facilitators of Treatment for Depression in a Latino Community: A Focus Group Study." *Community Mental Health Journal* 48, no. 1: 114–26.

US Census Bureau. 2015. "American Community Survey: Detailed Languages Spoken at Home and Ability to Speak English for the Population 5 Years and Over: 2009–2013." https://www.census.gov/topics/population/language-use/data.html.

US Census Bureau. 2016. "American Community Survey 5-Year Estimates (2012–2016)." https://www.census.gov/acs/www/data/data-tables-and-tools/data-profiles/2016/.

US Census Bureau. 2017. Retrieved March 3, 2018, from https://data.census.gov/cedsci/profile?g=1600000US0682954.

US Census Bureau. 2018. "Quick Facts: Visalia City, California." https://www.census.gov/quickfacts/fact/table/visaliacitycalifornia/POP815217#POP815217 (accessed April 12, 2019).

US Department of Health and Human Services. 2000. *Healthy People 2010: With Understanding and Improving Health and Objectives for Improving Health*. Washington, DC: US Government Printing Office.

Valdés, Guadalupe. 1982. "Social Interaction and Code-Switching Patterns: A Case Study of Spanish-English Alternation." In *Spanish in the United States: Sociolinguistics Aspects*, edited by Jon Amastae and Lucía Elías-Olivares, 209–29. Cambridge: Cambridge University Press.

Valdés, Guadalupe. 1988. "The Language Situation of Mexican Americans." In *Language Diversity*, edited by Sandra Lee McKay and Sau-ling Cynthia Wong, 111–39. San Francisco: Newbury House.

Van Leeuwen, Theo. 2008. *Discourse and Practice: New Tools for Critical Discourse Analysis*. New York: Oxford University Press.

Vickers, Caroline H., Ryan Goble, and Sharon K. Deckert. 2015. "Third Party Interaction in the Medical Context: Code-Switching and Control." *Journal of Pragmatics* 84: 154–71. https://doi.org/10.1016/j.pragma.2015.05.009.

Villa, Daniel J. 2010. "¿¡ Cómo Que Spanglish!? Creating a Service Learning Component for a Spanish Heritage Language Program." In *Building Communities and Making Connections*, edited by Susana Rivera-Mills and Juan Antonio Trujillo, 120–35. Newcastle upon Tyne: Cambridge Scholars.

Wallerstein, Nina, Bonnie Duran, John G. Oetzel, and Meredith Minkler, eds. 2017. *Community-Based Participatory Research for Health: Advancing Social and Health Equity*. San Francisco: Wiley.

Wassertheil-Smoller, Sylvia, Elva Arredondo, JianWeb Cai, Sheila F. Castaneda, James P. Choca, Linda C. Gallo, Molly Jung, Lisa M. LaVange, Elizabeth T. Lee-Ray, Thomas Mosley Jr., Frank J. Penedo, D. A. Santistaban, and P. C. Zee. 2014. "Depression, Anxiety, Antidepressant Use, and Cardiovascular Disease among Hispanic Men and Women of Different National Backgrounds: Results from the Hispanic Community Health Study/Study of Latinos." *Annals of Epidemiology* 24, no. 11: 822–30.

West, Candace. 1984. *Routine Complications: Troubles with Talk between Doctors and Patients*. Bloomington: Indiana University Press.

Wodak, Ruth. 1996. *Disorders of Discourse*. London: Longman.

Yellowlees, Peter M., Alberto Odor, Michelle Burke Parish, Ana-Maria Iosif, Karen Haught, and Donald Hilty. 2010. "A Feasibility Study of the Use of Asynchronous Telepsychiatry for Psychiatric Consultations." *Psychiatric Services* 61, no. 8: 838–40.

Yellowlees, Peter M., Alberto Odor, Kesha Patrice, Michelle Burke Parish, Najia Nafiz, Ana-Maria Iosif, and Donald Hilty. 2011. "Brief Communication Disruptive Innovation: The Future of Healthcare?" *Telemedicine and e-Health* 17, no. 3: 231–34.

Youdelman, Mara K. 2008. "The Medical Tongue: U.S. Laws and Policies on Language Access." *Health Affairs* 27, no. 2: 424–33.

Zentella, Ana Celia. 1997. *Growing Up Bilingual: Puerto Rican Children in New York*. Malden, MA: Blackwell.

Zuvekas, Samuel H., and Gregg S. Taliaferro. 2003. "Pathways to Access: Health Insurance, the Health Care Delivery System, and Racial/Ethnic Disparities, 1996–1999." *Health Affairs* 22, no. 2: 139–53. http://dx.doi.org/10.1377/hlthaff.22.2.139.

INDEX

abstract, 13, 14, 17, 23, 32, 35, 36–37, 107

affect, 68, 76, 86; analysis of, 78–79; concept of, 77–78; levels of, 76 fig. 3; verbal, 41

Ainsworth-Vaughn, Nancy, 81, 82, 84

alignment strategy, 62, 99; biased questions as, 116–21

Altarriba, Jeanette, 93

alternatives, 70, 75, 87, 110, 117n3; culturally meaningful, 76

ambiguity, space for, 110

anxiety, 86, 95, 100, 110; decreasing, 56; describing, 73; patient descriptions of, 74 table 4

aseguranza, 90, 91

assessments, 28, 79; psychiatric, 47, 82

assimilation, 41, 92

authority, 56, 79

behavior, 121; communicative, 76; culturally significant, 61–62; disrespectful, 63; socially undesirable, 71; substantiating, 62, 64

biases: implicit, 10, 21, 118, 119, 120, 121. *See also* questions, biased

bilingualism, 14, 17, 89, 90, 98, 104; code-switching and, 103

bonding: interpersonal, 105; masculinity and, 64

brain surgery, 32, 33, 95

bushes, *como* (like) as, 110–14

Caffi, Claudia, 110

California Healthcare Interpreting Association (CHIA), 9

Camarero, Garachana, 116n2

cancer, xii–xiii, 1, 2, 95, 125, 136; breast, xi–xii; kidney, 96

Carlat, Daniel J., 25, 37–38, 41, 50, 71

Central Valley, 15, 24, 41; health care workers in, 16–17; Spanish language in, 16–17

chapulines, story about, 54, 56

checking, tags and, 101–2

CLAS. *See* culturally and linguistically appropriate services

Clinton, Bill, 1

code-switching, 3, 12, 19, 104, 105, 106, 129, 134; bilingual speakers and, 103; categories for, 94, 94 table 9; contextual, 94–99;

doctor and patient, 94 table 9; elaboration/definition of, 99–101; medical terms and, 95–96; misconception about, 103; stigmatized view of, 96; translanguaging and, 89–90; using, 93–94, 98–99

colloquialisms, 3, 14, 17, 20, 50, 61, 69, 71, 75, 77, 82, 86, 129, 131; adopting, 74; listed, 72 table 3; purpose of, 87; using, 70, 72–73, 89

Colon, Eduardo, 5–6

communication, xi, 25, 30, 67, 68; assistance in, 8, 135; breakdown in, 51, 98; class and, 10; contextual, 136; doctor-patient, 11, 128, 130; effective, 66; examples of, 9; formal, 19; gender-based, 16; health care, 3, 4, 9–11, 137, 138; improving, 9–10, 20; interpersonal, 18, 21, 65; interpreted-mediated, 9–11; linguistics and, 4, 137; medical, 66, 80; transcultural, 3–4, 7, 12, 13, 19, 40, 45, 47, 54, 64, 65, 127, 128, 129, 132

communities, 23; of color, 138; knowledge of, 128; Latino, 24; marginalized, 138; Spanish-speaking, 20; voice for, 138

como, multifunctional uses of, 110–14

complications, 32–33, 35–36, 38–39, 39–40

compliments, 18, 50, 52; giving, 57–58, 65, 66, 133

confianza, 11, 14, 21, 86, 87, 105, 126, 132, 133, 134; creating, 18, 71, 89, 91, 96–97, 122, 127, 129; cultural construct of, 104; defined, 8; disrupting, 130; negotiating, 13

confirmation checks, 116, 118

consultations, 15, 65, 66, 131; face-to-face, 136; language-concordant, 126; questions for, 81; virtual, 136; words per, 83, 84 table 6

contact, 68, 83, 86, 90, 106; aural, 70; described, 76–77; language, 11; visual, 70

context, 94, 98–99, 103, 136; cultural, 68, 80; social, 86; sociopolitical, 80

conversations, 30, 43, 49; informal, 71; social, 52

Cordella, Marissa, 11, 31, 81, 83

Coupland, Justine, 49

cultural barriers, xi, 4, 24, 41, 125, 130, 136; addressing, 7–9, 137

cultural competency, 2, 7, 9, 10

cultural constructs, 8–9, 14 fig. 1, 137; Latino, 9, 19; synthesizing, 132–34

cultural differences, xi, 8, 9

cultural expectations, 51, 65, 122

cultural issues, 6; health care and, 7

cultural negotiations, 44

cultural systems, knowledge of, 4

culturally and linguistically appropriate services (CLAS), 7, 8

culture, xiv, 9, 17, 20, 51, 70, 73, 105; doctor-patient, 3, 11–12; dominant, 136; health care and, 12; interviews and, 23; language and, 7; minority-group, 20; multiple, 19

Curcó, Carmen, 116n2

De la Torre, Adela, 7, 74

definition, code-switching, 99–101

deformándolos, 92, 93

depression, 36, 42, 61, 71, 86, 110; colloquial terminology for, 73; describing, 73; patient descriptions of, 74 table 4; stigmatization of, 6; symptoms of, 6

desesperada/o, 33

diabetes, 2, 110, 127, 136

diagnosis, 5, 25, 27, 38, 52, 83, 97

Diagnostic and Statistical Manual of Mental Disorders: DSM-IV, 26, 97

dialect, 7, 91, 92; English-language, 128; using, 72–73

discourse, xiv, 18, 23, 45, 46, 82, 89, 127; doctor-patient, 11–12; interview, 67–68; markers, 31, 101, 102; medical, 10, 13, 45; spoken, 103

discourse analysis, 3, 4, 11, 17, 46, 135, 137

discrimination, 5, 41, 51; layers of, 126

doctors, 31, 32, 138; code-switching by, 94 table 8, 94 table 9, 97; Hispanic, 7; interruptions by, 84–85, 85 table 7; raising awareness for, 8

drugs, 3, 55, 71, 110

Dynamic Consultations: A Discourse Analytical Study of Doctor-Patient Communication, The (Cordella), 11

education, 5, 15, 16, 65, 79, 92; bilingual, 102; levels of, 4, 6, 15, 70, 137; medical, 127, 128–29

Eggins, Suzanne, 23, 55, 57, 62, 107

elaboration, code-switching, 99–101

empathy, showing, 41, 51

emphasis, adding, 102–3

English as a second language, 59

English language, xi; command of, 5; as dominant language, 67; influence of, 15, 106; limited proficiency in, 1

Erzinger, Sharry, 84

Estrada, Antonio L., 7

ethics, 10, 55, 126

ethnicity, 5n2, 16, 122, 136; language and, 4; questions and, 82

ethnographic studies, 93, 129

evaluation, 33, 36, 39, 40, 63, 64

familiarity, 4, 20, 41, 66, 71, 131

feedback, 70, 138

first-person plural, 59

floor, holding, 82–86

Flores, Yvette, 6, 73

Flores-Ferrán, Nydia: on mitigating devices, 108

Flynn, Patricia M., 51

Foreign Languages and Higher Education: New Structures for a Changed World (Modern Language Association), 19

formality: interlocutors and, 75–76; level of, 68, 69, 70, 75–76

Frankel, Richard, 81

García, Ofelia, 18

gender, 16, 63, 128; cultural constructs of, 137; identity, 137

genre, 12, 13, 14 fig. 1, 18, 26, 65; concrete, 68; conventions, 30; interview, 82; small talk, 52; social values and, 24; story, 45; subgenres and, 23; theory, 17, 24–25

genre analysis, 23, 24–25, 26, 65, 66, 68

gossip, 18, 52, 65, 133; agreeing with, 66; using, 61–64

grammar, 37, 109, 117, 118, 127; nonstandard, 71

greetings, 26–27, 28

Gumperz, John: classifications by, 93

Halliday, M. A. K., 2, 67

Hayes-Bautista, David, 50

health beliefs, cultural attunement to, 6

health care, xiii, 15, 17, 20, 65, 83, 104, 127, 134; advice on, 136; barriers to, 4, 138; communities in, 135; *confianza* in, 126;

continuity of, 51; culture and, 7, 12; decisions regarding, 119; disparities in, 8, 17, 51, 87, 129; effective, 24, 105; equity in, 8; follow-up, 126; improving, 136, 137; language and, 4–7, 137–38; Latino, 51; miscommunication in, 1; mistrust in, 125; patient-centered, 135; primary/preventive, 5; quality of, xiv, 3, 21; underrepresentation in, 138

Health Care Language Assistance Act (SB 853), 1–2

health care professionals. *See* medical practitioners

health issues, 2, 4, 12, 35, 37, 127; communication about, 3, 7; minority-language speakers and, 6; risk for, 125; talking about, 129

health literacy, 6, 80, 136

history, 126; developmental, 26; medical, 25, 26, 32, 35, 148–49, 150–51, 153–54; political, 4; psychiatric, 26; social, 4, 26, 37–38; sociodevelopmental, 4, 25, 37–41, 45, 122, 149–50, 154; sociopolitical, 3

HIV/AIDS, 2, 108, 125, 136

humor, 3, 17, 18, 52, 133; social norms and, 55; transcultural understanding and, 56; using, 55–57, 65, 66

illnesses, 136; history of, 30–37, 144–48

immigrants, 5, 55, 130; conversing with, xiii; rural, 47, 79

"Improving Access to Services for Persons with Limited English Proficiency" (Executive Order 13166), 1–2

informality, 3, 17, 70, 71, 76, 76 fig. 3, 77, 80, 87, 133

information, 4, 6, 81, 123, 136; collecting, 30, 87; confirming, 18, 115, 116, 117, 119; conveying, 7, 66; demographic, 29–30, 38, 52, 84, 144; medical, 49, 121; semantic loosening of, 121

instruction, 28, 29, 42; language, 138

interactions, 9, 34–35, 84, 115, 126, 134; doctor-patient, 4, 11–12, 14, 17, 20, 41, 45, 50, 80, 90, 132, 134, 135; English-language, 12, 67; frequency of, 77; health, 4, 12, 109; improving, 49; interpersonal, 5, 20, 21, 43, 65, 133; interpreter-mediated, 2; language, 23; medical, 7, 49, 108, 123, 132, 133, 136; psychiatric, 65; small talk, 65; social, 8, 50, 52; Spanish-language, 2, 135; symmetrical, 71; transcultural, 51 interlocutors, 13, 49, 67, 68, 81, 86, 107; affect and, 77, 78; formality and, 75–76; interrupting, 18; power of, 76; questions by, 79; relationship between, 45, 77, 82–83; social role of, 105

interpersonal, 12, 13, 17–18, 28, 107

interpretation, 28, 29, 42, 116; cultural, 74–75; selective, 10; space for, 116

interpreters, 2; ethnographic study of, 10; insights for, 21, 46–47, 66, 87, 105–6, 122–23; training, 9; value of, 10

interrogatives, biased, 117, 120, 121

interruptions, 82–86; minimizing, 84, 86; number of, 84–85; power and, 79, 83; respeto and, 84

interviews, 5n2, 21, 30, 35, 44, 45, 59, 60, 64, 83, 86, 115, 126; complete/sample of, 143–56; culture and, 23; genre of, 82, 119; medical, 46, 65, 84, 108; motivational, 12; procedure of, 28–29, 144; sections of, 25; settings for, 14–17; small talk and, 66; Spanish-language, 46; transcultural, 137. See also psychiatric interviews

intimacy, social distance and, 76–77

Jacobson, Rodolfo, 94, 95

jargon, using, 18, 50, 68

joking, 50, 54, 56

knowledge, 4, 10; colloquial, 75, 87, 135; cultural, 2, 3, 53, 87; folkloric, 75, 86; medical, 79; sociopolitical, 2, 3; transcultural, 2, 3, 17, 25, 46, 116, 122, 126, 127, 131, 137

Koike, Dale, 117n3

Labov, William, 35, 45

language, xi, 14 fig. 1, 128, 130; accommodations, 45, 91, 104, 134; assistance, 8, 10, 104; bilingual/misunderstanding, 106; choices, 123, 135; culture and, 7; ethnicity and, 4; everyday, 68–69; formal, 76 fig. 3; health care and, 4–7; ideational, 45; informal, 3, 17, 70, 76 fig. 3; interpersonal, 3, 4, 18, 105; lexical/grammatical role of, 12; medical, 68; minority-group, 20, 50; non-English, 93; patient, 46, 128; preferred, 133; repertoire, 89; role of, 25; symbolic value of, 2; use/understanding, 13; varieties in, 19–20, 21, 135

language barriers, 4, 5, 41, 104, 125; facing, 137; patient care and, 10

language metafunctions, 13, 13 table 1

like, multifunctional uses of, 110–14

linguistic analysis, 12–14, 20, 23

linguistics, xiv, 2, 9, 16, 17, 18, 20, 25, 80, 87, 93, 103, 104–5, 128, 129, 136; health communication and, 4

loanwords, 90, 91–92, 106

macrolanguage, 17, 51

marginalization, 41, 122, 126, 131, 138

Martin, James R., 35

Martínez, Glenn A., 9; on interpretation, 10; linguistic gradient and, 6; public health workers and, 104

masculinity, bonding and, 64

meaning-making, 73, 117, 134

medical practitioners, 20, 119, 121; distance of, 41; Hispanic, 7; insights for, 17, 21, 46–47, 66, 87, 105–6, 122–23; shortage of, 16–17; values and, 8. See also doctors

medical terms, 10, 21, 68; code-switching and, 95–96

medications, 6, 26, 110, 118

mental health, 5, 42, 68, 87, 134, 136; examinations, 26; inquiring about, 32

mental health care, 15, 131, 135; global, 90; Hispanic, 7; receiving, 6; resources, 17

metaphors, 97, 98, 137

Mini-International Neuropsychiatric Interview, 26

miscommunication, xii, 1, 135

misunderstandings, 74–75, 137

modality devices, 19, 108, 110, 121, 122, 123, 136; using, 109, 113. See also verbal modality

Modern Language Association, 19

narratives, 35, 38, 43, 60, 61, 80; complications in, 37; elaborate, 30; health, 4, 17; using, 46

negative polarity, 85, 116, 116n1, 117, 117n3, 118, 119, 120, 132, 133

nervios, 33, 73, 110

orientation, 28, 29, 30, 32, 34, 35, 38, 60

Ortega, Pilar, 90, 104, 128

panic attacks, 81, 95, 99, 101

parece, using, 113

patients: bilingual, 18, 92, 95, 97, 101, 103, 104, 105, 133–34; code-switching by, 94 table 8, 94 table 9; empowering, 66; interruptions and, 84–85, 85 table 7; passivation of, 119; private-practice, 80; talking by, 83

personal advice, 18, 52, 129, 133; giving, 58–59, 65, 66

personal exchanges, 29, 43, 65, 129, 132; described, 52–64

personalismo, 21, 50, 51, 54, 55, 61, 125, 132, 133; construct of, 65; defined, 8; negotiating, 13; showing, 57–58, 64, 105, 133; *simpatía* and, 14

positive statements, 55, 66

power, 82–86, 128; described, 79; distance, 18; dynamics, 17, 86, 108; gaps, 121, 133; inequality in, 86; interruptions and, 79, 83; migration, 121; mitigating, 89; questions and, 79–82; roles, 65, 108; social, 18; social distance and, 80; tenor and, 79

Poynton, Cate, 76

Prada, Josh, 90, 128

professional distance, maintaining, 41

pronouns, polite/informal, 19, 122

psychiatric disorders, 4, 25, 42, 58, 63, 77, 119, 132; screening for, 41, 4244, 154–56

Psychiatric Interview, The (Carlat), 26, 50

psychiatric interviews, 3, 4, 14, 21, 45, 46, 51–52, 65, 109, 110, 119, 121, 122, 127, 131, 133, 134; abstract levels of, 17; components of, 26, 27 table 2; field of, 68–70; genre of, 23–24, 26–44; holding floor in, 82; illness and, 30; linguistic options in, 86; medical perspectives on, 25; mode of, 70–75; power and, 79; questions for, 79, 80; register analysis of, 67; schematic structures of, 44; sections of, 25; small talk and, 27; sociodevelopmental questions of, 37; tenor of, 75–76; translanguaging and, 104; trust and, 105

questions, 42; analyzing, 117; asking, 18, 87; biased, 107, 116–21, 117n3, 133; consultation, 81; criteria for, 80–81; demographic, 85; descriptive statistics for, 81–82; doctor-patient, 67; ethnicity and, 82; patient, 33, 83 table 5; power and, 79–82; predetermined, 45; rhetorical, 80–81; sociodevelopmental, 37

racism, 6, 130

Ragan, Sandy L., 49

rapport, building, 42, 122

Rastogi, Mudita, 6

record of events, 30–31, 34, 60–61

recounts, 46, 52, 60–61, 65

regionalisms, 20, 71, 92

register, 12, 13, 14 fig. 1, 70, 76, 127, 135; analysis, 67, 68, 86; code-switching as, 92–94; formal, 4, 128; informal, 20, 128; intimate, 104; technical, 4, 68; variables, 13, 13 table 1

relationships: building, 77; clinical, 41; doctor-patient, 8, 83, 119; formal, 76; interpersonal, 17, 29, 52, 107, 108, 121, 122, 130, 134, 137; long-term, 80, 81; nonreciprocal-asymmetrical, 59; power, 68; social, 107; transcultural, 65

reorientation, 31, 34, 35, 61

resolution, 33, 36, 40

respeto, 21, 105, 122, 125, 132, 134; cultural rule of, 12; defined, 8; examples of, 19; interruptions and, 84; maintaining, 13, 70; showing, 14, 18, 86, 122, 127, 130, 133

responsibility, 108; displacing, 110, 121, 122

Rose, David, 35

Santiago-Rivera, Azara L., 93

schematic structures, 44, 45–46

screening, function of, 42–44

se me hace, using, 113

second-language learners, 19, 102

seguro médico, 90

self-disclosure, 3, 17, 52, 53, 58, 59–60, 61, 133; solidarity and, 59; using, 65, 66

self-image, 55, 121

semantic extension, 90, 91–92

sentirse subido, 97

service learning, 129

SFL. *See* systemic functional linguistics

Shea, Shawn Christopher, 82

short responses, 29, 31–32, 42–43, 54, 56, 58; deviations from, 44, 44 fig. 2, 45

simpatía, 11, 17, 21, 24, 30, 40, 47, 50, 105, 125, 132, 133; defined, 8; focus on, 12; knowledge of, 27; negotiating, 13; *personalismo* and, 14 skills, xi, 132; communication, 128, 137; interactional, 46; interpersonal, 51, 128; language, 3; literacy, 4; transcultural, 105

Slade, Diana, 55, 57, 62, 83

small talk, 3, 17, 27, 28, 61, 82, 125, 143–44, 151–53; boundaries of, 51–52; importance of, 66; life world and, 49; psychiatric interactions and, 65; term, 50; topics of, 59–60; using, 65, 89

social distance, 95; intimacy and, 76–77; power and, 80

social expectations, 2–3, 17

social norms, 55, 65

social roles, 41, 65, 105, 108, 118

social systems, knowledge of, 4

socialization, 3, 4, 20, 126

sociocultural perspective, 19, 70

sociodemographic profiles, 110

sociodevelopmental history, 4, 25, 37–41, 45, 122, 149–50, 154

socioeconomic backgrounds, 11, 30, 40, 127

sociolinguistic awareness, 2, 3, 4, 11, 65, 89, 90, 93, 104, 105, 126, 127–28, 131, 132, 135

solidarity, 52; bilingual, 101; building, 54, 62; communicating, 105; self-disclosure and, 59

Spanglish, 92

Spanish language, 9; formal, 20; immediacy of, 54; medical, 90, 128; Mexican, xiii, xiv, 116; as minority language, 67; professional, 19, 20; role of, 5; rural, 3, 20; speaking, xiii, 3, 4, 16–17; varieties in, xiii–xiv; working-class, 10

status, 79; financial, 37, 61, 80; social, 16, 19, 114; socioeconomic, 4, 6, 81, 87, 92, 137

strategies: discourse, 17, 24, 71, 121, 127, 129–32; interpersonal, 25; linguistic, 105; politeness, 18, 19, 107, 109, 122, 130; transcultural, 19, 24. See also alignment strategy

subgenres, 23, 26, 30, 31, 44, 45; emergence of, 24–25, 46; summary of, 27 table 2

substance abuse, 26, 148–49

superiority/inferiority distinction, 11, 21, 135

synonyms, standard, 72 table 3

systemic functional linguistics (SFL), 2, 12, 17, 51, 67, 77, 107, 108, 109, 110, 129, 134, 135; genre theory and, 24; as social theory, 13; using, 3

tags: checking and, 101–2; using, 114–16

Tardy, Christine M., 24

tenor, 75–76, 82–83; power and, 79

third-person focus, 62–63, 64

topics: cultural, 52–55; social, 49; task-oriented, 52

transcultural competence, 3–4, 12, 19, 21, 44, 45, 51, 65, 70, 73, 77, 82, 87, 90, 104–5, 109, 125, 127, 129; at linguistic level, 17; models of, 66

translanguaging, 18, 91, 91n1, 97, 131; as appropriate, 96; code-switching and, 89–90; practices, 95, 105–6; psychiatric interviews and, 104; space for, 104

translations, 21; direct, 97; multiple, 73n1

trust, 134; building, 27, 52, 104, 122; doctor-patient, 27; creating, 18, 105, 122; establishing, 122; mutual, 21

Valdés, Guadalupe, 92

values, 108; cultural, 3, 8, 12, 132; gender-role, 62; Latino, 8, 9, 19, 134; social, 20, 24

Van Leeuwen, Theo, 119

verbal modality, 107, 110–11, 120, 121, 122, 123; mitigation and, 108–9; using, 12. See also modality devices

vergüenza, 6, 58, 136

Waletzky, Joshua, 35, 45

West, Candace, 81

wrap-up, 63, 64

Zentella, Ana Celia, 93, 103

GLOBAL LATIN/O AMERICAS

FREDERICK LUIS ALDAMA AND LOURDES TORRES, SERIES EDITORS

This series focuses on the Latino experience in its totality as set within a global dimension. The series showcases the variety and vitality of the presence and significant influence of Latinos in the shaping of the culture, history, politics and policies, and language of the Americas—and beyond. It welcomes scholarship regarding the arts, literature, philosophy, popular culture, history, politics, law, history, and language studies, among others.

Building Confianza: *Empowering Latinos/as Through Transcultural Health Care Communication*
   DALIA MAGAÑA

Fictions of Migration: Narratives of Displacement in Peru and Bolivia
   LORENA CUYA GAVILANO

Baseball as Mediated Latinidad: Race, Masculinity, Nationalism, and Performances of Identity
   JENNIFER DOMINO RUDOLPH

False Documents: Inter-American Cultural History, Literature, and the Lost Decade (1975–1992)
   FRANS WEISER

Public Negotiations: Gender and Journalism in Contemporary US Latina/o Literature
   ARIANA E. VIGIL

Democracy on the Wall: Street Art of the Post-Dictatorship Era in Chile
   GUISELA LATORRE

Gothic Geoculture: Nineteenth-Century Representations of Cuba in the Transamerican Imaginary
   IVONNE M. GARCÍA

Affective Intellectuals and the Space of Catastrophe in the Americas
   JUDITH SIERRA-RIVERA

Spanish Perspectives on Chicano Literature: Literary and Cultural Essays
   EDITED BY JESÚS ROSALES AND VANESSA FONSECA

Sponsored Migration: The State and Puerto Rican Postwar Migration to the United States
   EDGARDO MELÉNDEZ

La Verdad: An International Dialogue on Hip Hop Latinidades
   EDITED BY MELISSA CASTILLO-GARSOW AND JASON NICHOLS

CPSIA information can be obtained
at www.ICGtesting.com
Printed in the USA
LVHW042307020122
707496LV00001B/10